WORKBOOK TO ACCOMPANY

COMPREHENSIVE MEDICAL TERMINOLOGY

WORKBOOK TO ACCOMPANY

COMPREHENSIVE MEDICAL TERMINOLOGY

Fifth Edition

Betty Davis Jones, MA, RN, CMA (AAMA)

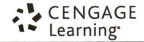

CENGAGE
Learning

Australia • Brazil • Mexico • Singapore • United Kingdom • United States

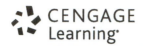

Workbook to Accompany Comprehensive Medical Terminology, Fifth Edition
Betty Davis Jones

SVP, GM Skills & Global Product Management:
  Dawn Gerrain

Product Director: Matthew Seeley

Senior Director, Development:
  Marah Bellegarde

Product Development Manager: Juliet Steiner

Product Manager: Laura Stewart

Senior Content Developer:
  Debra M. Myette-Flis

Product Assistant: Deborah Handy

Vice President, Marketing Services:
  Jennifer Ann Baker

Marketing Manager: Jonathan Sheehan

Senior Production Director: Wendy Troeger

Production Director: Andrew Crouth

Content Project Manager: Thomas Heffernan

Managing Art Director: Jack Pendleton

Cover image(s): ©iStockPhoto.com/angelhell

Library of Congress Control Number: 2015933403

ISBN: 978-1-305-07463-7

Cengage Learning
20 Channel Center Street
Boston, MA 02210
USA

Cengage Learning is a leading provider of customized learning solutions with employees residing in nearly 40 different countries and sales in more than 125 countries around the world. Find your local representative at **www.cengage.com**

Cengage Learning products are represented in Canada by Nelson Education, Ltd.

To learn more about Cengage Learning, visit **www.cengage.com**

Purchase any of our products at your local college store or at our preferred online store **www.cengagebrain.com**

Notice to the Reader
Publisher does not warrant or guarantee any of the products described herein or perform any independent analysis in connection with any of the product information contained herein. Publisher does not assume, and expressly disclaims, any obligation to obtain and include information other than that provided to it by the manufacturer. The reader is expressly warned to consider and adopt all safety precautions that might be indicated by the activities described herein and to avoid all potential hazards. By following the instructions contained herein, the reader willingly assumes all risks in connection with such instructions. The publisher makes no representations or warranties of any kind, including but not limited to, the warranties of fitness for particular purpose or merchantability, nor are any such representations implied with respect to the material set forth herein, and the publisher takes no responsibility with respect to such material. The publisher shall not be liable for any special, consequential, or exemplary damages resulting, in whole or part, from the readers' use of, or reliance upon, this material.

Printed at CLDPC, USA, 03-20

CONTENTS

This workbook is designed as a tool to help you learn. It is intended to accompany *Comprehensive Medical Terminology,* Fifth Edition, by Betty Davis Jones. A variety of exercises are included to help you master key concepts in each chapter of the text. Exercises include labeling, build-a-word, find the term, completion, word elements and common abbreviation matching, spelling, *What Is This?*, scenarios, and *Putting It All Together.* The workbook to accompany the fifth edition of the text includes additional learning exercises such as construct-a-word, pronunciation to spelling, *Match Point,* and *Is It the Same?*

The *Review Checkpoint* feature in your text correlates to the exercises in this workbook. Each time you see a Review Checkpoint in your text, stop and complete the related exercises in the workbook to measure how well you understand the material studied in the text.

The workbook exercises for Chapters 1–4 are designed to reinforce the terms presented in those chapters. Exercises for these chapters include build-a-word, completion, word element matching, and spelling. Beginning with Chapter 5, the Review Checkpoint follows major sections in your text. The workbook exercises are designed to help you assess your mastery of the content before you move on to the next section of the textbook chapter. After you have read each major section in the chapter, stop and complete the related Review Checkpoint exercises to *check* your understanding of the material. If you have trouble answering the workbook questions at the end of a section, go back and reread that section of text.

Chapters 5–17, following the *Putting It All Together* section, include labeling exercises to assist you in learning the major structures in each body system. The labeling exercises and several other exercises involve written answers. Writing out the answers helps you absorb more information and boosts your learning. Additional learning exercises have been added to these chapters to provide more opportunities to improve the learner's understanding of medical terms.

WORKBOOK TO ACCOMPANY

COMPREHENSIVE MEDICAL TERMINOLOGY

Word-Building Rules

REVIEW CHECKPOINT

A. Completion

Read each statement carefully and write the appropriate answer in the space provided.

1. The word root is defined as _____.

2. A suffix is defined as _____.

3. A combining form is defined as a(n) _____.

4. A compound medical word is made up of the following three elements: _____.

5. The combining vowels most often used to join a word root to a suffix are _____ and _____.

6. A prefix is defined as _____.

7. The definition of a medical word begins with defining the _____ first, and continuing to "read" backward through the word as you define it.

8. When a medical word has a prefix, the definition of the word usually begins with defining the _____ first, the _____ second, and the word root(s) last.

9. A(n) _____ is a name for a disease, organ, procedure, or body function that is derived from the name of a person.

10. A word cannot end with this word element: _____; the word must end with a suffix.

B. Matching

Match the terms on the left with the correct definition on the right.

_____ 1. combining form   a. compound word

_____ 2. attaches to beginning of word   b. word root + vowel

_____ 3. suffix   c. word root

_____ 4. combining form + word root + suffix   d. prefix

_____ 5. basic foundation of a word   e. word ending

C. Completion

Read each statement carefully and write the appropriate answer in the space provided.

1. A _____ is placed at the beginning of the word (applies always).

2. A _____ is placed at the end of the word (applies always).

3. The use of more than one _____ in a word creates the need for combining vowels to connect the roots.

4. The definition of a medical word usually begins with defining the suffix first and continuing to "read" _____ through the word as you define it.

5. When a medical word has a prefix, the definition of the word usually begins with defining the _____ first, the prefix second, and the root(s) last.

D. Matching

Match the terms on the left with the correct definition on the right.

_____ 1. words beginning with the "f" sound   a. Word may begin with *ps, c*.

_____ 2. words beginning with the "k" sound   b. Word may begin with *pn, kn*.

_____ 3. words beginning with the "n" sound   c. Word may begin with *ph*.

_____ 4. words beginning with the "s" sound   d. Word may begin with *ge, gi, gy*.

_____ 5. words beginning with the "j" sound   e. Word may begin with *c, ch, qu*.

Prefixes

REVIEW CHECKPOINT

A. Build-a-Word

Test your word building skills. Using the clues below, build the appropriate medical terms.

1. Build a word that means "without breathing."

   _____ + __pnea_____ = _____

   prefix   suffix   word

2. Build a word that means "the study of life."

   _____ + __logy_____ = _____

   prefix   suffix   word

3. Build a word that means "paralysis of one side (half) of the body."

   _____ + __plegia_____ = _____

   prefix   suffix   word

4. Build a word that means "between the ribs."

   _____ + __cost____ + __al_____ = _____

   prefix   word root   suffix   word

5. Build a word that means "within a vein."

   _____ + __ven_____ + __ous_____ = _____

   prefix   word root   suffix   word

6. Build a word that means "slow heartbeat."

   _____ + __card____ + __ia_____ = _____

   prefix   word root   suffix   word

7. Build a word that means "slightly bluish, grayish, slatelike, or dark discoloration of the skin."

   _____ + ___o_____ + __derm____ + __a_____ = _____

   prefix   combining vowel   word root   suffix   word

8. Build a word that means "instrument used to look inside the body."

   _____ + __scope_____ = _____

   prefix   suffix   word

9. Build a word that means "less than normal blood oxygen level."

$$\underline{\hspace{4cm}}_{\text{prefix}} + \underline{\hspace{3cm}\text{ox}\hspace{3cm}}_{\text{word root}} + \underline{\hspace{3cm}\text{emia}\hspace{3cm}}_{\text{suffix}} = \underline{\hspace{4cm}}_{\text{word}}$$

10. Build a word that means "rapid heartbeat."

$$\underline{\hspace{4cm}}_{\text{prefix}} + \underline{\hspace{3cm}\text{card}\hspace{3cm}}_{\text{word root}} + \underline{\hspace{3cm}\text{ia}\hspace{3cm}}_{\text{suffix}} = \underline{\hspace{4cm}}_{\text{word}}$$

B. Matching

Match the terms on the left with the correct definition on the right.

_____ 1. ad-		a. green
_____ 2. alb-		b. toward, increase
_____ 3. auto-		c. self
_____ 4. chlor/o		d. against
_____ 5. contra-		e. white
_____ 6. exo-		f. between
_____ 7. inter-		g. all
_____ 8. intra-		h. outside, outward
_____ 9. pan-		i. around
_____ 10. peri-		j. within

C. Completion

Read each statement carefully and write the appropriate answer in the space provided.

1. The prefix *ecto-* means _____

2. The prefix *eu-* means _____

3. The prefix *exo-* means _____

4. The prefix *hetero-* means _____

5. The prefix *hydro-* means _____

6. The prefix *mono-* means _____

7. The prefix *tri-* means _____

8. The prefix *semi-* means _____

9. The prefix *trans-* means _____

10. The prefix *pre-* means _____

D. Spelling

Identify the correct spelling of each medical term. Write the correct spelling in the space provided.

1. pseudo-   psudo-   _____

2. quadra-   quadri-   _____

3. reub-   rube-   _____

4. xanth/o   zanth/o   _____

5. meso-   mezzo-   _____

6. tachy-   tacky-   _____

7. pery-   peri-   _____

8. multe-   multi-   _____

9. ambi-   ambe-   _____

10. brady-   bradi-   _____

CHAPTER 3

Suffixes

REVIEW CHECKPOINT

A. Completion

Read each statement carefully and write the appropriate answer in the space provided.

1. The suffix that means "embryonic stage of development" is _____.

2. The suffix that means "blood condition" is _____.

3. The suffix that refers to pregnancy is _____.

4. The suffix that means "stretching or dilation, as in stretching or dilation of the stomach," is

   _____.

5. The suffix that means "seizure, or attack," is _____.

6. The suffix that means "sensitivity to pain" is _____.

7. The suffix that means "swelling or herniation" is _____.

8. The suffix that means "pain" is _____.

9. The suffix that means "an instrument used to record" is _____.

10. The suffix that means "record or picture" is _____.

B. Matching

Match the terms on the left with the correct definition on the right.

_____ 1. -mania   a. stone

_____ 2. -metry   b. the process of measuring

_____ 3. -lytic   c. condition

_____ 4. -ism   d. a mental disorder; a "madness"

_____ 5. -lith   e. destruction

_____ 6. -megaly   f. surgical fixation

_____ 7. -oid   g. enlargement

_____ 8. -plegia   h. condition

_____ 9. -osis   i. paralysis

_____ 10. -pexy   j. resembling

C. Spelling

Identify the correct spelling of each medical term. Write the correct spelling in the space provided.

1. -oma   -omah   _____

2. -phobea   -phobia   _____

3. -ptosis   -tosis   _____

4. -rrhagia   -rrhaghia   _____

5. -trispy   -tripsy   _____

6. -penia   -penea   _____

7. -rrhexus   -rrhexis   _____

8. -osis   -osus   _____

9. -lisis   -lysis   _____

10. -side   -cide   _____

D. Build-a-Word

Test your word building skills. Using the clues below, build the appropriate medical terms.

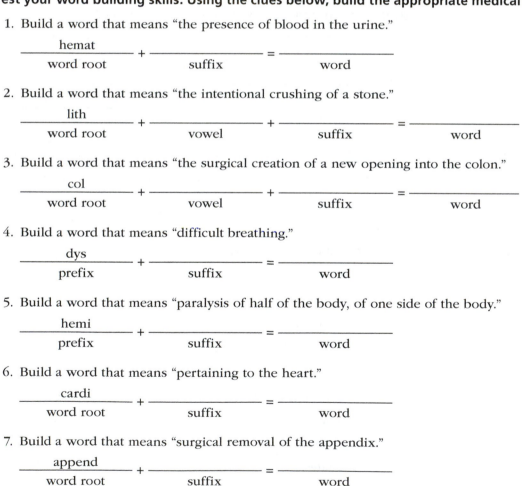

1. Build a word that means "the presence of blood in the urine."

    $\dfrac{\text{hemat}}{\text{word root}}$ + $\dfrac{}{\text{suffix}}$ = $\dfrac{}{\text{word}}$

2. Build a word that means "the intentional crushing of a stone."

    $\dfrac{\text{lith}}{\text{word root}}$ + $\dfrac{}{\text{vowel}}$ + $\dfrac{}{\text{suffix}}$ = $\dfrac{}{\text{word}}$

3. Build a word that means "the surgical creation of a new opening into the colon."

    $\dfrac{\text{col}}{\text{word root}}$ + $\dfrac{}{\text{vowel}}$ + $\dfrac{}{\text{suffix}}$ = $\dfrac{}{\text{word}}$

4. Build a word that means "difficult breathing."

    $\dfrac{\text{dys}}{\text{prefix}}$ + $\dfrac{}{\text{suffix}}$ = $\dfrac{}{\text{word}}$

5. Build a word that means "paralysis of half of the body, of one side of the body."

    $\dfrac{\text{hemi}}{\text{prefix}}$ + $\dfrac{}{\text{suffix}}$ = $\dfrac{}{\text{word}}$

6. Build a word that means "pertaining to the heart."

    $\dfrac{\text{cardi}}{\text{word root}}$ + $\dfrac{}{\text{suffix}}$ = $\dfrac{}{\text{word}}$

7. Build a word that means "surgical removal of the appendix."

    $\dfrac{\text{append}}{\text{word root}}$ + $\dfrac{}{\text{suffix}}$ = $\dfrac{}{\text{word}}$

8. Build a word that means "surgical repair of the nose."

<u>   rhin   </u> + <u>   o   </u> + <u>   </u> = <u>   </u>

    word root   combining vowel   suffix   word

9. Build a word that means "one who takes or records X-rays."

<u>   radi   </u> + <u>   o   </u> + <u>   graph   </u> + <u>   </u> = <u>   </u>

    word root   combining vowel   word root   suffix   word

10. Build a word that means "difficult breathing."

<u>   dys   </u> + <u>   </u> = <u>   </u>

    prefix   suffix   word

Whole Body Terms

REVIEW CHECKPOINT

A. Completion

Read each statement carefully and write the appropriate answer in the space provided.

1. The semipermeable barrier that is the outer covering of a cell is known as the cell _____.

2. The gel-like substance that surrounds the nucleus of a cell is the _____.

3. The tissue that covers the internal and external organs of the body and lines the vessels, body cavities, glands, and body organs is known as _____ tissue.

4. The _____ plane divides the body into front and back portions.

5. The largest and strongest of the vertebrae of the spinal column, located in the lower back, are known as the _____ vertebrae.

6. The body cavity that contains the urinary bladder and the reproductive organs is the _____ cavity.

7. The fifth segment of the vertebral column, also known as the tail bone, is known as the _____.

8. The standard reference position for the body as a whole is known as _____ position.

9. The term that means "pertaining to the front of the body" is _____.

10. The position of the body lying on the abdomen, facedown is _____.

B. Matching

Match the terms on the left with the correct definition on the right.

_____ 1. intervertebral disc

_____ 2. long axis

_____ 3. McBurney's point

_____ 4. proximal

_____ 5. sacrum

_____ 6. thoracic cavity

_____ 7. abdominal cavity

_____ 8. spinal cavity

_____ 9. ventral cavity

a. located on the right side of the abdomen, about about two-thirds of the distance between the umbilicus and the anterior bony prominence of the hip

b. the singular triangular-shaped bone that results from the fusion of five individual bones of the child

c. toward or nearest the trunk of the body, or nearest to the point of origin of a body part

d. a flat, circular platelike structure of cartilage that serves as a cushion (or shock absorber) between the vertebrae

e. essentially the midline of the body

f. liver, gallbladder, spleen, stomach, pancreas, intestines, and kidneys

____ 10. cranial cavity

g. brain

h. lungs, heart, aorta, esophagus, and trachea

i. nerves of the spinal cord

j. organs on the front side of the body

C. Spelling

Identify the correct spelling of each medical term. Write the correct spelling in the space provided.

1. chromasomes   chromosomes   _____

2. histolagist   histologist   _____

3. nucleus   neuclus   _____

4. umbilicul   umbilical   _____

5. visceral   viscerul   _____

6. superior   superier   _____

7. dysplasia   dysplasea   _____

8. naval   navel   _____

9. mediol   medial   _____

10. peritoneum   peritineum   _____

D. Build-a-Word

Test your word building skills. Using the clues below, build the appropriate medical terms.

1. Build a word that means "pertaining to the front; belly side."

   _____ + _____ = _____
   word root   suffix   word

2. Build a word that means "pertaining to the spine."

   _____ + _____ = _____
   word root   suffix   word

3. Build a word that means "pertaining to the middle and side of a structure."

   _____ + _____ + _____ + _____ = _____
   word root   vowel   word root   suffix   word

4. Build a word that means "pertaining to the side."

   _____ + _____ = _____
   word root   suffix   word

5. Build a word that means "a medical scientist who specializes in the study of tissues."

   _____ + _____ + _____ = _____
   word root   vowel   suffix   word

6. Build a word that means "pertaining to the skull."

   _____ + _____ = _____
      word root   suffix   word

7. Build a word that means "the study of cells."

   _____ + _____ + _____ = _____
      word root   combining vowel   suffix   word

8. Build a word that means "pertaining to the area over or upon the stomach."

   _____ + _____ + _____ = _____
      prefix   word root   suffix   word

9. Build a word that means "pertaining to the back."

   _____ + _____ = _____
      word root   suffix   word

10. Build a word that means "pertaining to the internal organs."

   _____ + _____ = _____
      word root   suffix   word

Labeling

Labeling 1

Using the structure names listed below, label the following illustration of component parts of a cell by writing your answers in the spaces provided.

Mitochondrion

Cell membrane

Lysosome

Ribosome

Nucleus

Cytoplasm

1. _____

2. _____

3. _____

4. _____

5. _____

6. _____

(continued)

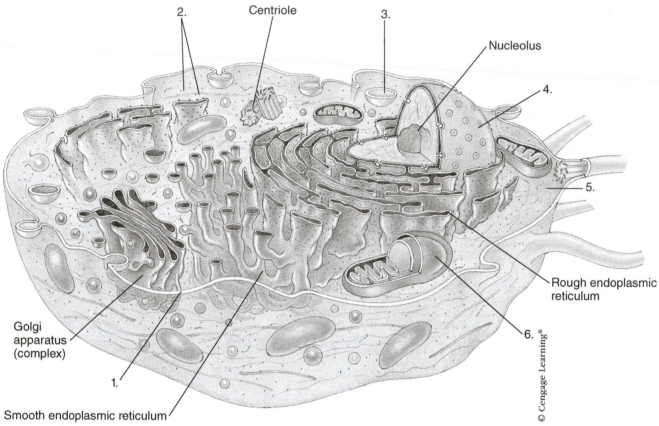

Component parts of a cell

Labeling 2

Using the terms listed below, label the following illustration of abdominal quadrants by writing your answers in the spaces provided.

Left upper quadrant (LUQ)

Right upper quadrant (RUQ)

Left lower quadrant (LLQ)

Right lower quadrant (RLQ)

7. _____

8. _____

9. _____

10. _____

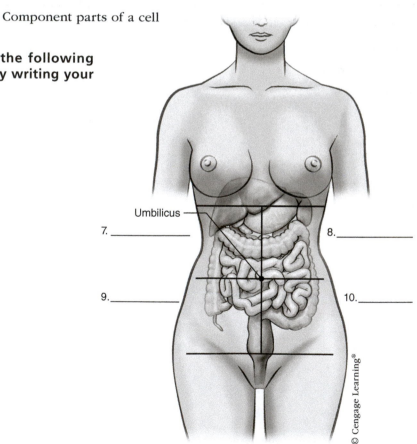

Abdominal quadrants

CHAPTER 5

The Integumentary System

A. Review Checkpoint: Anatomy & Physiology

Completion: Read each statement carefully and write the appropriate answer in the space provided.

1. The outer layer of the skin that contains no blood or nerve supply is the _____.

2. The cells that provide color to the skin and some protection from the harmful effects of the ultraviolet rays of the sun are the _____.

3. The dermis, the inner thick layer of skin lying directly beneath the epidermis, is also known as the _____.

4. The oil glands are also known as the _____ glands.

5. The sudoiferous gland is also known as the _____ gland.

B. Review Checkpoint: Vocabulary

Build-a-Word: Test your word building skills. Using the clues below, build the appropriate medical terms.

1. Build a word that means "a condition of blueness."

   _____ + _____ = _____
   word root   suffix   word

2. Build a word that means "one who specializes in the study of the skin."

   _____ + _____ + _____ = _____
   word root   combining vowel   suffix   word

3. Build a word that means "inflammation of the skin."

   _____ + _____ = _____
   word root   suffix   word

4. Build a word that means "destruction of the nail (separation of a fingernail from its bed, beginning at the free margin)."

   _____ + _____ + _____ = _____
   word root   combining vowel   suffix   word

5. Build a word that means "drainage, or flow, of sebum."

   _____ + _____ + _____ = _____
   word root   combining vowel   suffix   word

C. Review Checkpoint: Word Elements

Matching: Match the word elements listed on the left to the appropriate definition on the right.

_____	1. adip/o	a.	yellow
_____	2. hidr/o	b.	nails
_____	3. onych/o	c.	tissue
_____	4. xanth/o	d.	fat
_____	5. hist/o	e.	sweat

D. Review Checkpoint: Skin Lesions

Matching: Match the lesions listed on the left to the appropriate definition on the right.

_____ 1. abrasion

_____ 2. blister

_____ 3. laceration

_____ 4. boil

_____ 5. wheal

a. a circumscribed, slightly elevated lesion of the skin that is paler in the center than its surrounding edges

b. a tear in the skin; a torn, jagged wound

c. furuncle

d. a scraping or rubbing away of the skin or mucous membrane as a result of friction to the area

e. vesicle

E. Review Checkpoint: Pathological Conditions

Completion: Read each statement carefully and write the appropriate answer in the space provided.

1. A contagious, superficial skin infection characterized by serous vesicles and pustules filled with millions of staphylococcus or streptococcus bacteria, usually forming on the face, is known as _____.

2. Seborrheic keratosis appears as brown or waxy yellow wart-like lesion(s), 5 to 20 mm in diameter, loosely attached to the skin. It is also known as _____.

3. Another name for a nevus is a(n) _____.

4. A highly contagious parasitic infestation caused by the "human itch mite," resulting in a rash, pruritus, and slightly raised thread-like skin lines is known as _____.

5. A verruca is also known as a(n) _____.

F. Review Checkpoint: Diagnostic Techniques, Treatments, and Procedures

Completion: Read each statement carefully and write the appropriate answer in the space provided.

1. A noninvasive treatment that uses subfreezing temperature to freeze and destroy the tissue is known as _____.

2. Removal of debris, foreign objects, and damaged or necrotic tissue from a wound to prevent infection and to promote healing is known as _____.

3. The removal or destruction of tissue with an electrical current is known as _____.

4. Aspiration of fat through a suction cannula or curette to alter the body contours is known as _____.

5. An incision made into the necrotic tissue resulting from a severe burn, "incision into a scab," is known as a(n) _____.

G. Review Checkpoint: Common Abbreviations

Matching: Match the abbreviations on the left with the correct definition on the right.

____ 1. bx   a. ointment

____ 2. ID   b. intradermal

____ 3. SLE   c. biopsy

____ 4. ung.   d. purified protein derivative

____ 5. PPD   e. systemic lupus erythematosus

H. Review Checkpoint: Putting It All Together

The following questions offer a review of the material studied in the integumentary system. Read each question carefully and select, or write, the most appropriate answer.

1. A thin-walled skin lesion containing clear fluid is known as a(n)

   a. blister
   b. ulcer
   c. polyp
   d. wheal

2. Thin flakes of hardened epithelium that are shed from the epidermis are known as

   a. vesicles
   b. polyps
   c. scales
   d. hives

3. A common inflammatory disorder seen on the face, chest, back, and neck and appearing as papules, pustules, and comedos is known as

   a. acne vulgaris
   b. scabies
   c. callus
   d. eczema

4. An enlarged, irregularly shaped, and elevated scar that forms due to the presence of large amounts of collagen during the formation of the scar is known as a

   a. nevus
   b. burn
   c. keloid
   d. callus

5. Herpes zoster is also known as _____.

6. Onychomycosis is a fungal infection of the _____.

7. A highly contagious parasitic infestation caused by blood-sucking lice is known as _____.

8. A gradual thickening of the dermis and swelling of the hands and feet to a state in which the skin is anchored to the underlying tissue is known as _____.

9. Tinea is more commonly known as _____.

10. A skin biopsy, in which the complete tumor or lesion is removed for analysis, is known as a(n) _____ biopsy.

11. A skin biopsy, in which a small specimen of tissue in the "cookie cutter" fashion is removed, is known as a(n) _____ biopsy.

12. A small, flat discoloration of the skin that is neither raised nor depressed is known as a

    a. callus
    b. polyp

    c. macule
    d. nodule

13. A small, stalk-like growth that protrudes upward or outward from a mucous membrane surface—resembling a mushroom stalk—is known as a

    a. callus
    b. polyp

    c. mole
    d. nodule

14. An abnormal passageway between two tubular organs (such as the rectum and vagina) or from an organ to the body surface is known as a

    a. fistula
    b. bulla

    c. comedo
    d. carbuncle

15. A large blister is also called a

    a. fistula
    b. comedo

    c. bulla
    d. carbuncle

16. A modified sweat gland that lubricates the skin of the ear canal with yellowish-brown waxy substance called cerumen (or earwax) is known as a(n) _____ gland.

17. A crack-like sore or groove in the skin or mucous membrane is known as a(n) _____.

18. The process of scraping material from the wall of a cavity or other surface for the purpose of removing abnormal tissue or unwanted material is known as

    a. curettage
    b. diaphoresis

    c. electrodessication
    d. excoriation

19. Inflammation of the fold of skin surrounding the fingernail, also called runaround, is known as

    a. petechial
    b. pimple

    c. paronychia
    d. pachyderma

20. A cyst filled with a cheesy material consisting of sebum and epithelial debris that has formed in the duct of a sebaceous gland, also known as an epidermoid cyst, is known as a(n) _____ cyst.

I. Labeling

Labeling 1

Using the structure names listed below, label the following diagram of the structure of the hair by writing your answers in the spaces provided.

Hair follicle

Bulb

Root of hair

Shaft of hair

Epidermis

1. _____

2. _____

3. _____

4. _____

5. _____

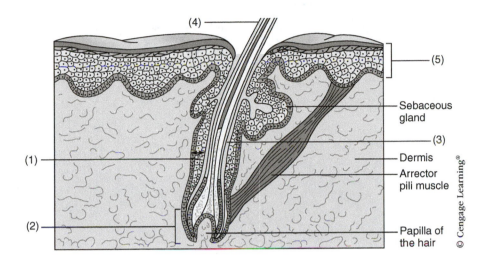

Labeling 2

Using the structure names listed below, label the following illustration of glands of the skin by writing your answers in the spaces provided.

Pore

Subcutaneous layer

Sweat gland

Epidermis

Dermis

Sebaceous gland

1. _____

2. _____

3. _____

4. _____

5. _____

6. _____

(continued)

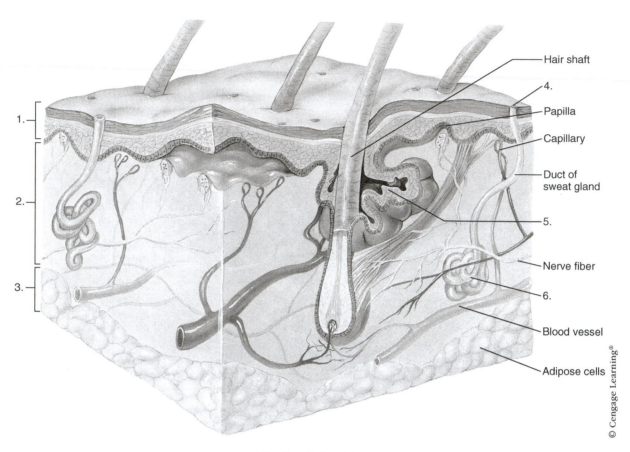

Hair shaft

4.

Papilla

Capillary

Duct of
sweat gland

5.

Nerve fiber

6.

Blood vessel

Adipose cells

© Cengage Learning®

1.

2.

3.

Glands of the skin

J. What Is This?

Read the statements that follow and identify the diagnostic technique, treatment, or procedure described. Write the appropriate answer in the space provided.

1. Dr. Delgato has scheduled Ms. Smith for a noninvasive treatment procedure that uses subfreezing temperature to freeze and destroy the tissue. He will be removing a basal cell carcinoma from the side of her face. A local anesthetic will be applied to the surface of the lesion, followed by the application of liquid nitrogen, which freezes and destroys the tumor tissue. What is the name of this procedure?

_____

2. Mr. Hill received severe burns on his left leg when trying to put out an uncontrolled brush fire in the woods adjacent to his house. He is receiving periodic treatments for the burns and has to undergo periodic treatments that involve removal of debris and damaged or necrotic tissue from the burn to prevent infection and to promote healing. This treatment is usually followed by hydrotherapy to assist in the healing of the burns. What is this procedure?

_____

3. There is one area on Mr. Hill's leg that had a full-thickness burn. The physician made an incision into the necrotic tissue that resulted from this severe burn to remove the necrotic tissue in order to prevent a wound infection of the burn site. The incision into the scar relieves the tightness in the affected area and allows for expansion of tissue created by swelling and aids in the healing process. What is the name of this procedure?

_____

4. When Mr. Hill's third-degree burn area on his leg did not heal well, his physician decided to perform a surgical procedure that involved placing tissue on Mr. Hill's burn site to provide the protective mechanisms of skin to the area that was unable to regenerate skin. The tissue was taken from another part of Mr. Hill's body. What is the name of this procedure? (hint: two words)

_____

5. Dr. Thompson suspects that his patient, Jimmy, has head lice. To confirm his diagnosis, he will place Jimmy in a darkened room and shine an ultraviolet light on the affected area. If the fungal spores are present, they will appear a brilliant, fluorescent blue-green color. What type of lamp will Dr. Thompson use for this procedure?

_____

K. Spelling

Identify the correct spelling of each medical term. Write the correct spelling in the space provided.

1. absess   abscess   _____
2. cysk   cyst   _____
3. fissure   fisher   _____
4. pruritus   pruritis   _____
5. lesion   lesian   _____

L. Pronunciation to Spelling

Using the phonetic pronunciations that follow, spell the words correctly. Write your response in the space provided.

1. (am-pew-**TAY**-shun) _____
2. (**KAR**-bung-kul) _____
3. (kon-**TOO**-shun) _____
4. (**dye**-ah-foh-**REE**-sis) _____
5. (**sub**-kew-**TAY**-nee-us) _____

M. Construct-a-Word

Using the word elements below, construct words that match the definitions provided. Write your answer in the space provided.

epi-	cutane/o	-ous
pachy-	cyan/o	-osis
	dermat/o	-logist
	derm/o	-is
	derm/o	-a

1. pertaining to the skin _____

2. a condition of blueness _____

3. a physician who specializes in the treatment of diseases and disorders of the skin _____

4. the outermost layer of the skin _____

5. abnormal thickening of the skin _____

CHAPTER 6

The Skeletal System

A. Review Checkpoint: Anatomy & Physiology

Completion: Read each statement carefully and write the appropriate answer in the space provided.

1. The thick, white fibrous membrane that covers the surface of the long bone, except at joint surfaces, is known as the _____.

2. The first seven pairs of ribs—attached to the sternum in the front and to the vertebrae in the back—are known as the _____ ribs.

3. The main shaft-like portion of a long bone is known as the _____.

4. The layer of cartilage that separates the diaphysis from the epiphysis of the bone, which provides the means for the bone to increase in length during childhood, is known as the _____ plate/line.

5. The conversion of fibrous connective tissue and cartilage into bone or a bony substance is known as _____.

B. Review Checkpoint: Vocabulary

Build-a-Word: Test your word-building skills. Using the clues below, build the appropriate medical terms.

1. Build a word that means "pertaining to between the ribs."

   _____ + _____ + _____ = _____
      prefix   word root   suffix   word

2. Build a word that means "a condition of narrowing"—an abnormal condition characterized by a narrowing or restriction of an opening or passageway in a body structure.

   _____ + _____ = _____
      word root   suffix   word

3. Build a word that means "a mature bone cell."

   _____ + _____ + _____ = _____
      word root   combining vowel   suffix   word

4. Build a word that means "pertaining to the neck."

   _____ + _____ = _____
      word root   suffix   word

5. Build a word that means "formation of blood"; the normal formation and development of blood cells in the bone marrow.

   _____ + _____ + _____ = _____
      word root   combining vowel   suffix   word

C. Review Checkpoint: Word Elements

Matching: Match the word elements listed on the left to the appropriate definition on the right.

_____ 1. cost/o   a. crooked, bent

_____ 2. calcane/o   b. ribs

_____ 3. malac/o   c. upper jaw

_____ 4. maxill/o   d. heel bone

_____ 5. scoli/o   e. softening

D. Review Checkpoint: Pathological Conditions

Completion: Read each statement carefully and write the appropriate answer in the space provided.

1. A condition in which bones that were once strong become fragile due to loss of bone density (porous bones) is known as _____.

2. A local or generalized infection of the bone and bone marrow, resulting from a bacterial infection that has spread to the bone tissue through the blood, is known as _____.

3. The most common benign bone tumor that literally means "tumor of the cartilage and bone" and that usually involves the femur and the tibia is known as a(n) _____.

4. The medical term for an abnormally outward curvature of a portion of the spine, commonly known as humpback or hunchback, is _____.

5. A fracture that occurs as a result of a force so great that it splinters or crushes a segment of the bone is known as a(n) _____ fracture.

E. Review Checkpoint: Diagnostic Techniques, Treatments, and Procedures

Completion: Read each statement carefully and write the appropriate answer in the space provided.

1. The treatment for a fracture that consists of aligning the bone fragments through manual manipulation or traction, without making an incision into the skin, is known as a(n) _____ (hint: two words)

2. The process of removing a small sample of bone marrow from a selected site with a needle for the purpose of examining the specimen under a microscope is known as a bone marrow _____

3. The treatment for a fracture that consists of realigning the bone under direct observation during surgery is known as a(n) _____ (hint: two words)

4. Devices such as screws, pins, wires, and nails may be used to internally maintain the bone alignment while healing takes place. These devices, more commonly used with fractures of the femur and fractures of joints, are known as _____ (hint: three words)

5. The dual energy X-ray absorptiometry (DEXA) is a noninvasive procedure that measures bone _____

F. Review Checkpoint: Common Abbreviations

Matching: Match the abbreviations on the left with the correct definition on the right.

_____	1. THR	a.	sacrum
_____	2. TMJ	b.	fracture
_____	3. Fx	c.	total hip replacement
_____	4. TKR	d.	temporomandibular joint
_____	5. S1	e.	total knee replacement

G. Review Checkpoint: Putting It All Together

The following questions offer a review of the material studied in the skeletal system. Read each question carefully and select, or write, the most appropriate answer.

1. The bone that forms the forehead and the upper part of the bony cavities that contain the eyeballs is the

   a. temporal bone
   b. frontal bone
   c. occipital bone
   d. parietal bone

2. The bone that forms the back of the head and the base of the skull (the back portion of the floor of the cranial cavity) is the

   a. temporal bone
   b. frontal bone
   c. occipital bone
   d. parietal bone

3. The two bones that form the upper jaw are known as the

   a. maxillary bones
   b. temporal bones
   c. parietal bones
   d. zygomatic bones

4. The two bones, one on each side of the face, that form the high part of the cheek and the outer border of the eye orbits are known as the

   a. mandibular bones
   b. maxillary bones
   c. zygomatic bones
   d. nasal bones

5. The second segment of the vertebral column, consisting of 12 vertebrae that connect with the 12 pairs of ribs, are identified as

   a. cervical vertebrae
   b. thoracic vertebrae
   c. lumbar vertebrae
   d. sacrum

6. The medical term for the tail bone is the _____.

7. The upper arm bone is known as the _____.

8. The lower arm bone on the lateral, or thumb side, of the arm is the _____.

9. The lower arm bone on the medial, or little finger, side of the arm is the _____.

10. The bones of the wrist are known as the _____.

11. The term that refers to the bony ring formed by the hip bones is

    a. pelvic girdle
    b. ilium
    c. iliac crest
    d. symphysis pubis

12. The thigh bone is known as the

    a. fibula
    b. tibia
    c. femur
    d. patella

13. The knee bone, or kneecap, is called the

    a. patella   c. tibia
    b. femur   d. tarsals

14. The larger and stronger of the two lower leg bones, also known as the shin bone, is the

    a. fibula   c. patella
    b. tibia   d. femur

15. The space between the bones of an infant's cranium—"soft spot"—is known as a

    a. foramen   c. fontannelle
    b. fissure   d. condyle

16. An opening or hollow space in a bone—a cavity within a bone—is called a

    a. sinus   c. tubercle
    b. tuberosity   d. suture

17. An abnormal inward curvature of a portion of the spine, commonly known as swayback, is called _____.

18. An abnormal lateral (sideward) curvature of a portion of the spine is known as _____.

19. A fracture that occurs when a bone, weakened by a preexisting disease, breaks in response to a force that would not cause a normal bone to break is known as a

    a. hairline fracture   c. pathological fracture
    b. Colles' fracture   d. comminuted fracture

20. A fracture that occurs at the lower end of the radius, within 1 inch of connecting with the wrist bones, is known as a

    a. hairline fracture   c. pathological fracture
    b. Colles' fracture   d. comminuted fracture

H. Labeling

Labeling 1

Using the structure names listed below, label the following illustration of cranial bones by writing your answers in the spaces provided.

Mandible

Occipital bone

Frontal bone

Temporal bone

Maxilla

1. _____

2. _____

3. _____

4. _____

5. _____

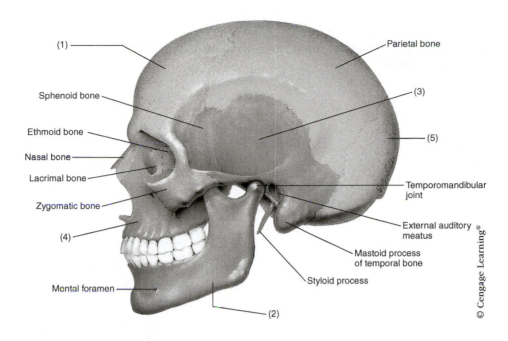

Labeling 2

Using the structure names listed below, label the following illustration of a long bone by writing your answers in the spaces provided.

Proximal epiphysis

Spongy bone (marrow)

Distal epiphysis

Diaphysis

Yellow marrow

1. _____

2. _____

3. _____

4. _____

5. _____

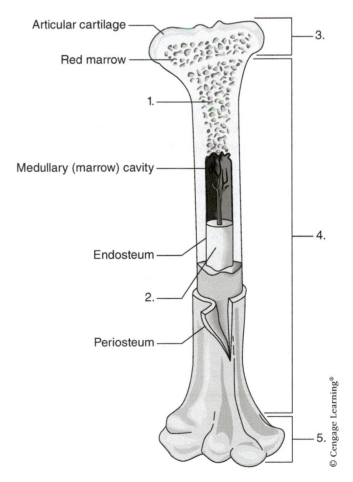

Structure of a long bone

Labeling 3

Using the structure names listed below, label the following illustration of facial bones by writing your answers in the spaces provided.

Vomer bone

Mandible

Zygomatic bone

Nasal bone

Lacrimal bone

Maxillae

1. _____

2. _____

3. _____

4. _____

5. _____

6. _____

Facial bones

Labeling 4

Using the structure names listed below, label the following illustrations of fractures by writing your answers in the spaces provided.

Impacted fracture

Greenstick (incomplete) fracture

Colles' fracture

Open (compound, complete) fracture

Comminuted fracture

Closed (simple, complete) fracture

1. _____

2. _____

3. _____

4. _____

5. _____

6. _____

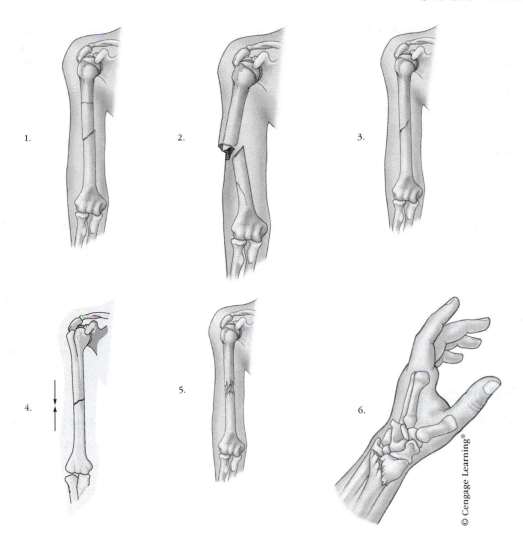

1.

2.

3.

4.

5.

6.

© Cengage Learning®

I. What Is This?

Read the statements that follow and identify the diagnostic technique, treatment, or procedure described. Write the appropriate answer in the space provided.

1. Susan Black fell and sustained a simple fracture of her left arm. The doctor in the emergency room will align the bone fragments through manual manipulation or traction, without making an incision into the skin. What type of maneuver is this?

   _____

2. Jim Queen was injured in an automobile accident and sustained a compound fracture of his right femur. The orthopedic surgeon will realign the bone under direct observation during surgery. What type of surgery is this?

   _____

3. When the surgeon is performing the surgery on Jim Queen, he decides to insert screws into the neck of the femur to internally maintain the bone alignment while healing takes place. What are these devices called?

   _____

4. The physician suspects that Julie Carson is suffering from anemia. To assist him in his diagnosis, he has ordered a test that involves the process of removing a small sample of bone marrow from a selected site with a needle for the purpose of examining the specimen under a microscope. What procedure is this?

_____

5. Maria Gonzales, age 56, is scheduled for her yearly physical today. One of the tests the physician will order is a noninvasive procedure that measures bone density. What is the abbreviation for this exam?

_____

J. Spelling

Identify the correct spelling of each medical term. Write the correct spelling in the space provided.

1. condyle   condole   _____

2. periostum   periosteum   _____

3. stenosus   stenosis   _____

4. mandibular   mandibuler   _____

5. palatine   palantine   _____

K. Pronunciation to Spelling

Using the phonetic pronunciations that follow, spell the word correctly. Write your response in the space provided.

1. (**pair**-ee-**AH**-stee-um) _____

2. (**CAR**-tih-laj) _____

3. (**FISH**-ur) _____

4. (**OSS**-tee-oh-sites) _____

5. (trah-**BEK**-yoo-lay) _____

L. Construct-a-Word

Using the word elements listed, construct a word that matches the definition provided. Write your answer in the space provided.

inter-	cervic/o	-al
peri-	oste/o	-poiesis
	cost/o	-al
	oste/o	-um
	hemat/o	-blast

1. pertaining to the neck _____

2. the formation and development of blood cells in the bone marrow _____

3. pertaining to between the ribs _____

4. the thick, white, fibrous membrane that covers the surface of a long bone _____

5. immature bone cell that actively produces bony tissue _____

CHAPTER 7

Muscles and Joints

A. Review Checkpoint: Anatomy & Physiology

Completion: Read each statement carefully and write the appropriate answer in the space provided.

1. Muscles that operate under conscious control are known as _____ muscles.

2. The triangular-shaped muscle that extends across the back of the shoulder, covers the back of the neck, and inserts on the clavicle and scapula is the _____ muscle.

3. The muscle that is used when biting and chewing, is located at the angle of the jaw, and raises the mandible and closes the jaw, is known as the _____ muscle.

4. A joint in which the bones have a space between them called the joint cavity that is lined with synovial membrane is called a(n) _____ joint.

5. A joint that allows movement in many directions around a central point and has a ball-shaped head that fits into the concave depression of another bone is known as a(n) _____.

B. Review Checkpoint: Vocabulary

Build-a-Word: Test your word building skills. Using the clues below, build the appropriate medical terms.

1. Build a word that means "pertaining to the cheek."

   _____ + _____ = _____
       word root   suffix   word

2. Build a word that means "pertaining to the chest" (other than thoracic).

   _____ + _____ = _____
       word root   suffix   word

3. Build a word that means "pertaining to a joint."

   _____ + _____ = _____
       word root   suffix   word

4. Build a word that means "surgical repair of a joint."

   _____ + _____ + _____ = _____
       word root   vowel   suffix   word

5. Build a word that means "inflammation of a bursa."

   _____ + _____ = _____
       word root   suffix   word

C. Review Checkpoint: Word Elements

Matching: Match the word elements listed on the left to the appropriate definition on the right.

_____ 1. arthr/o   a. surgical puncture

_____ 2. -graphy   b. surgical repair

_____ 3. oste/o   c. process of recording

_____ 4. -plasty   d. bone

_____ 5. -centesis   e. joint

D. Review Checkpoint: Pathological Conditions

Completion: Read each statement carefully and write the appropriate answer in the space provided.

1. An abnormal enlargement of the joint at the base of the great toe, in which the great toe deviates laterally, causing it to either override or undercut the second toe is known as hallux valgus or a(n) _____.

2. A disease that is an acute recurrent inflammatory infection transmitted through the bite of an infected deer tick is known as _____ disease.

3. Degenerative joint disease is also known as _____.

4. A group of genetically transmitted disorders characterized by progressive symmetrical wasting of skeletal muscles, with no evidence of nerve involvement or degeneration of nerve tissue, that has an onset early in life is known as _____. (hint: two words)

5. An injury to the body of the muscle or attachment of the tendon resulting from overstretching, overextension, or misuse is known as a(n) _____.

E. Review Checkpoint: Diagnostic Techniques, Treatments, and Procedures

Completion: Read each statement carefully and write the appropriate answer in the space provided.

1. The process of recording the strength of the contraction of a muscle when it is stimulated by an electric current is known as _____.

2. The extraction of a specimen of muscle tissue, through either a biopsy needle or an incisional biopsy, for the purpose of examining it under a microscope is known as a(n) _____. (hint: two words)

3. The surgical puncture of a joint with a needle for the purpose of withdrawing fluid for analysis is known as a(n) _____.

4. The process of X-raying the inside of a joint, after a contrast medium has been injected into the joint, is known as _____.

5. The surgical reconstruction (repair) of a joint is a(n) _____.

F. Review Checkpoint: Common Abbreviations

Matching: Match the abbreviations on the left with the correct definition on the right.

_____ 1. EMG   a. rheumatoid arthritis

_____ 2. OA   b. electromyography

_____ 3. RF   c. intramuscular

_____ 4. IM   d. osteoarthritis

_____ 5. RA   e. rheumatoid factor

G. Review Checkpoint: Putting It All Together

The following questions offer a review of the material studied in the chapter on muscles and joints. Read each question carefully and select, or write, the most appropriate answer.

1. Muscle fibers are held together by thin sheets of fibrous connective tissue called

   a. fascia
   b. tendons

   c. ligaments
   d. cartilage

2. The point of attachment of the muscle to the bone it moves is called the

   a. platysma
   b. insertion

   c. origin
   d. triceps

3. The muscle located above and near the ear is the

   a. masseter
   b. buccinators

   c. trapezius
   d. temporal

4. The large, fan-shaped muscle that crosses the upper part of the front of the chest, originating from the sternum and crossing over the humerus and forming the anterior border of the axilla (armpit), is the

   a. trapezius
   b. pectoralis major

   c. biceps brachii
   d. latissimus dorsi

5. The point of attachment of a muscle to a bone that is less movable (i.e., the more fixed end of attachment) is the

   a. platysma
   b. insertion

   c. origin
   d. triceps

6. Muscles that attach to the bones of the skeleton, also known as striated muscle, are known as _____ muscles.

7. Muscles found in the walls of hollow organs and tubes such as the stomach, intestine, respiratory passageways, and blood vessels, also known as visceral muscles, are known as _____ muscles.

8. Muscles that have a striped appearance when viewed under a microscope, such as skeletal and cardiac muscles, are known as _____ muscles.

9. Muscles that operate under conscious control, such as those responsible for movement of the face, eyes, tongue, and pharynx, are under _____ control.

10. Movement of a bone toward the midline of the body is known as _____.

11. Movement of a bone away from the midline of the body is known as _____.

12. The act of turning the palm of the hand up or forward, as if you were receiving change from a cashier, is known as

    a. pronation
    b. supination

    c. rotation
    f. dorsiflexion

13. A small sac that contains synovial fluid for lubricating the area around the joint where friction is most likely to occur is known as a

    a. bunion
    b. bursa

    c. kyphosis
    d. suture

14. An immovable joint is called a

    a. bunion
    b. bursa

    c. kyphosis
    d. suture

15. A bending motion that decreases the angle between two bones is known as

    a. extension
    b. pronation

    c. flexion
    d. dorsiflexion

16. Bending the foot downward, at the ankle, as in ballet dancing is known as

    a. pronation
    b. dorsiflexion

    c. supination
    d. plantar flexion

17. Connective tissue bands that join bone to bone, offering support to the joint, are known as _____.

18. A tear in the muscles that form a "cuff" over the upper end of the arm (head of the humerus) is known as a(n) _____ cuff tear.

19. An abnormal enlargement of the joint at the base of the great toe is a

    a. bursa
    b. bunion

    c. contracture
    d. tendon

20. An injury to the body of the muscle or attachment of the tendon resulting from overstretching, overextension, or misuse is known as a

    a. strain
    b. sprain

    c. torn meniscus
    d. contracture

H. Labeling

Labeling 1

Using the terms listed below, label the following illustrations of movement of joints by writing your answers in the spaces provided.

Extension

Rotation

Adduction

Flexion

Abduction

1. _____

2. _____

3. _____

4. _____

5. _____

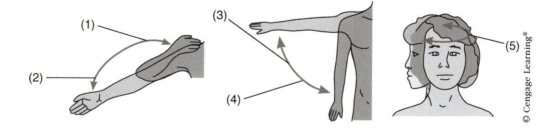

Labeling 2

Using the terms listed below, label the following illustrations of movement of joints by writing your answers in the spaces provided.

Plantar flexion

Circumduction

Supination

Dorsiflexion

Pronation

1. _____

2. _____

3. _____

4. _____

5. _____

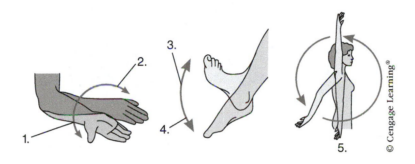

Labeling 3

Using the terms listed below, label the following illustration of muscles of the head and neck by writing your answers in the spaces provided.

Masseter

Buccinator

Sternocleidomastoid

Temporal

Zygomatic arch

1. _____

2. _____

3. _____

4. _____

5. _____

(continued)

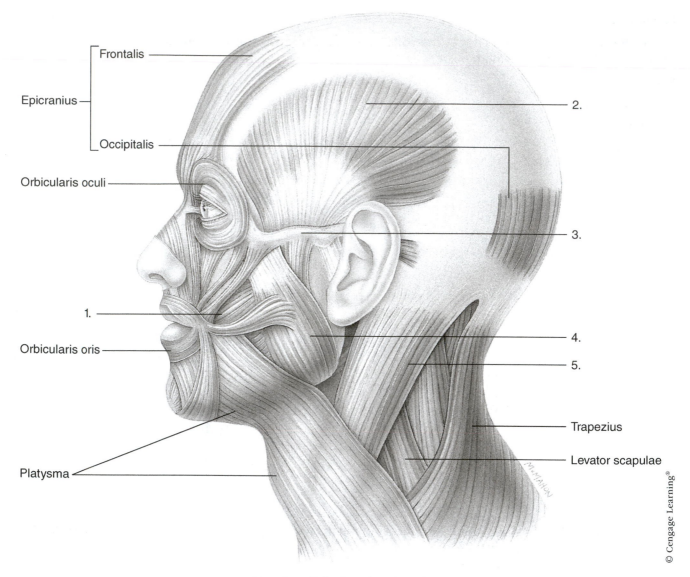

Frontalis

Epicranius

Occipitalis

Orbicularis oculi

1.

Orbicularis oris

Platysma

2.

3.

4.

5.

Trapezius

Levator scapulae

Muscles of the head and neck

I. What Is This?

Read the statements that follow and identify the diagnostic technique, treatment, or procedure described. Write the appropriate answer in the space provided.

1. Michael Jay injured his right knee in a basketball game two days ago. Since the injury, the knee has remained swollen and quite uncomfortable. Dr. Bone plans to do a procedure that involves the surgical puncture of the joint with a needle to withdraw the fluid from the joint for analysis. What is the name of this procedure?

   _____

2. Susan is a data-entry technician in her office and has noticed slight numbness in her wrist and progressive weakness in her ability to grasp things with her left hand. Dr. Tyler is performing a procedure that records the strength of the contraction of a muscle when it is stimulated by an electric current, to assist him in his diagnosis of Susan's condition. What is the name of this procedure?

   _____

3. Dr. Boggs suspects that Mr. Smith has muscular dystrophy and is checking for muscle atrophy. To examine the tissue under a microscope, she will perform a procedure that involves extraction of a specimen of muscle tissue through a biopsy needle. What is the name of this procedure? (hint: two words)

_____

4. Joe Timberlake injured his knee in a recent football championship game. His injury is severe enough that he has not been able to put any pressure on the knee for two days. The doctor has ordered a procedure that involves X-raying the joint—after a contrast medium has been injected into the joint—to determine the damage. What is the name of this procedure?

_____

5. The doctor suspects that Mrs. Payne has rheumatoid arthritis. He has ordered a blood test that measures the presence of unusual antibodies that develop in a number of connective tissue diseases, such as rheumatoid arthritis. What is the name of this test? (hint: two words)

_____

J. Spelling

Identify the correct spelling of each medical term. Write the correct spelling in the space provided.

1. suture   sucher   _____
2. malase   malaise   _____
3. atrophy   atropy   _____
4. buccinator   bucksinator   _____
5. trapesius   trapezius   _____

K. Pronunciation to Spelling

Using the phonetic pronunciations that follow, spell the word correctly. Write your response in the space provided.

1. (**FASH**-ee-ah) _____
2. (**STRY**-ay-ted) _____
3. (**AT**-roh-fee) _____
4. (**bun**-yun-**ECK**-toh-mee) _____
5. (**dor**-sih-**FLEK**-shun) _____

L. Construct-a-Word

Using the word elements that follow, construct a word that matches the definition provided. Write your answers in the space provided.

arthr/o	-algia
electr/o	-graphy
arthr/o	-ectomy
electr/o	-osis
my/o	-plasty
ganglion/o	
kyph/o	

1. pain in the joints _____

2. the process of recording the strength of the contraction of a muscle when it is stimulated by an electric current _____

3. surgical removal of a ganglion _____

4. another name for humpback _____

5. surgical repair of a joint _____

The Nervous System

A. Review Checkpoint: Anatomy & Physiology

Completion: Read each statement carefully and write the appropriate answer in the space provided.

1. A knot-like mass of nerve cell bodies located outside the central nervous system (CNS) is known as a(n) _____.

2. Nerves that carry impulses from the body to the central nervous system are known as _____ nerves.

3. The space between two nerves over which the impulse must cross is known as a(n) _____.

4. The three layers of protective membranes that surround the brain and spinal cord are known as the _____.

5. The largest part (and the uppermost portion) of the brain is the _____.

B. Review Checkpoint: Vocabulary

Build-a-Word: Test your word building skills. Using the clues below, build the appropriate medical terms.

1. Build a word that means "without sensitivity to pain."

   _____ + _____ = _____
   prefix   suffix   word

2. Build a word that means "difficult speech."

   _____ + _____ = _____
   prefix   suffix   word

3. Build a word that means "the study of muscle movement."

   _____ + _____ + _____ = _____
   word root   combining vowel   suffix   word

4. Build a word that means "inflammation of a nerve."

   _____ + _____ = _____
   word root   suffix   word

5. Build a word that means "paralysis of all four extremities (and the trunk of the body)."

   _____ + _____ = _____
   prefix   suffix   word

C. Review Checkpoint: Word Elements

Matching: Match the word elements listed on the left to the appropriate definition on the right.

_____ 1. brady-	a. seizure
_____ 2. kinesi/o	b. tension, tone
_____ 3. ton/o	c. slow
_____ 4. -lepsy	d. partial paralysis
_____ 5. -paresis	e. movement

D. Review Checkpoint: Pathological Conditions

Completion: Read each statement carefully and write the appropriate answer in the space provided.

1. A condition in which there is an absence of the brain and spinal cord at birth is known as _____.

2. A condition caused by a brief interruption of brain function, usually with a loss of consciousness lasting for a few seconds, is known as a cerebral _____.

3. Inflammation of the brain or spinal cord tissue largely caused by a virus that enters the central nervous system when the person experiences a viral disease such as measles or mumps or through the bite of a mosquito or tick is known as _____.

4. A syndrome of recurring episodes of excessive irregular electrical activity of the brain resulting in involuntary muscle movements called seizures is known as _____.

5. A chronic progressive neuromuscular disorder causing severe skeletal muscle weakness (without atrophy) and fatigue, which occurs at different levels of severity is known as _____.

   (hint: two words)

E. Review Checkpoint: Diagnostic Techniques, Treatments, and Procedures

Completion: Read each statement carefully and write the appropriate answer in the space provided.

1. A visualization of the cerebral vascular system via X-ray after the injection of a radiopaque contrast medium into an arterial blood vessel (carotid, femoral, or brachial) is known as a cerebral _____.

2. Measurement of electrical activity produced by the brain and recorded through electrodes placed on the scalp is termed _____.

3. The surgical removal of the bony arches from one or more vertebrae to relieve pressure from the spinal cord is known as a(n) _____.

4. The test used to evaluate cerebellar function and balance is the _____ test.

5. The introduction of contrast medium into the lumbar subarachnoid space through lumbar puncture in order to visualize the spinal cord and vertebral canal through X-ray examination is known as a(n) _____.

F. Review Checkpoint: Common Abbreviations

Matching: Match the abbreviation on the left with the correct definition on the right.

_____ 1. CNS   a. pneumoencephalogram

_____ 2. EMG   b. magnetic resonance imaging

_____ 3. MRI   c. multiple sclerosis

_____ 4. PEG   d. central nervous system

_____ 5. MS   e. electromyography

G. Review Checkpoint: Putting It All Together

The following questions offer a review of the material studied in the nervous system. Read each question carefully and select, or write, the most appropriate answer.

1. A small seizure in which there is a sudden temporary loss of consciousness lasting only a few seconds is known as a(n)

   a. aura
   b. absence seizure
   c. aneurysm
   d. cerebral contusion

2. The inability to convert one's thoughts into writing is known as

   a. agraphia
   b. agnosia
   c. alexia
   d. aphasia

3. A localized dilation in the wall of an artery that expands with each pulsation of the artery, usually caused by hypertension or atherosclerosis, is known as a(n)

   a. deficit
   b. axon
   c. aneurysm
   d. gyrus

4. A deep sleep in which the individual cannot be aroused and does not respond to external stimuli is known as (a)

   a. coma
   b. contusion
   c. concussion
   d. dementia

5. A projection that extends from the nerve cell body, which receives impulses and conducts them on to the cell body, is known as a(n)

   a. fissure
   b. synapse
   c. dendrite
   d. axon

6. A state of being sluggish is known as _____.

7. Another name for a nerve cell is a(n) _____.

8. The uppermost part of the brain stem is known as the _____.

9. A physician who specializes in treating the diseases and disorders of the nervous system is known as a(n) _____.

10. Paralysis of the lower extremities and trunk, usually due to spinal cord injuries, is known as _____.

11. The part of the peripheral nervous system that provides voluntary control over skeletal muscle contractions is known as the

   a. somatic nervous system
   b. central nervous system
   c. autonomic nervous system
   d. parasympathetic nervous system

12. A seizure characterized by the presence of muscle contraction or tension followed by relaxation, creating a "jerking" movement of the body, is known as a(n)

a. absence seizure
b. narcoleptic seizure
c. epileptic seizure
d. tonic-clonic seizure

13. A temporary or permanent unilateral weakness or paralysis of the muscles in the face following trauma to the face, an unknown infection, or a tumor pressing on the facial nerve rendering it paralyzed is known as

a. petit mal seizure
b. Bell's palsy
c. cerebral palsy
d. cerebrovascular accident

14. A small seizure in which there is a sudden temporary loss of consciousness lasting only a few seconds, also known as an absence seizure, is called a

a. petit mal seizure
b. Bell's palsy
c. cerebral palsy
d. cerebrovascular accident

15. A recurring, pulsating, vascular headache usually developing on one side of the head, which is characterized by a slow onset that may be preceded by an aura, is known as a

a. cluster headache
b. tension headache
c. migraine headache
d. sinus headache

16. The medical term for a headache is _____.

17. A collection of blood located above the dura mater and just below the skull is known as a(n) _____ hematoma.

18. A congenital disorder in which there is an abnormal increase of cerebrospinal fluid in the brain that causes the ventricles of the brain to dilate, resulting in an increased head circumference in the infant with open fontanels, is known as _____.

19. A rare syndrome of uncontrolled sudden attacks of sleep is known as _____.

20. An acute viral infection seen mainly in adults who have had chicken pox, characterized by inflammation of the underlying spinal or cranial nerve pathway (producing painful vesicular eruptions on the skin along these nerve pathways), is known as _____.

H. Labeling

Using the terms listed below, label the following illustration of the neuron by writing your answers in the spaces provided.

Dendrites

Axon

Cell body

Synapse

Nucleus

1. _____

2. _____

3. _____

4. _____

5. _____

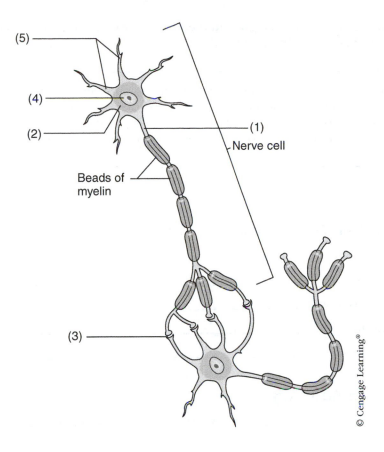

(5)

(4)

(2)

(1)
Nerve cell

Beads of
myelin

(3)

© Cengage Learning®

I. What Is This?

Read the statements that follow and identify the diagnostic technique, treatment, or procedure described. Write the appropriate answer in the space provided.

1. The doctor has ordered a procedure for Mr. Daze. This test involves the measurement of electrical activity produced by the brain and is recorded through electrodes placed on the scalp. The electrodes are connected to a machine that amplifies the electrical activity and records it on moving paper. What is the name of this procedure?

   _____

2. Mrs. Hertz has been suffering from chronic back pain for months. Her doctor has ordered a surgical procedure that is used to interrupt a portion of the sympathetic nerve pathway for the purpose of relieving chronic pain. What is the name of this procedure?

   _____

3. Pedro Gonzales has an order from his doctor to wear a TENS unit for his recurring sciatica. This is a form of cutaneous stimulation for pain relief that supplies electrical impulses to the nerve endings of a nerve close to the pain site. The electrodes are placed on the skin and connected to the stimulator by flexible wires. The electrical impulses are distinct enough to hinder the transmission of pain signals to the brain. What is the name of this procedure? (hint: four words)

   _____

4. Mrs. Falls is scheduled for a test to evaluate cerebellar function and balance. During this test, she will be asked to stand quietly with her feet together and hands at her sides—to attain equilibrium. Then she will be asked to close her eyes and maintain equilibrium without swaying or falling. She will then be

asked to lift her hands to shoulder height and then close her eyes without her hands drifting downward. What is the name of this test? (hint: two words)

_____

5. The doctor suspects that Tommy Smith has bacterial meningitis. She has ordered a test that involves the insertion of a hollow needle into the subarachnoid space, generally between the third and fourth lumbar vertebrae below the level of the spinal cord under strict aseptic technique, to withdraw cerebrospinal fluid for further examination. What is the name of this test? (hint: two words)

_____

J. Spelling

Identify the correct spelling of each medical term. Write the correct spelling in the space provided.

1. cephalalgia   cephalgia   _____

2. aura   auror   _____

3. kinesology   kinesiology   _____

4. jyrus   gyrus   _____

5. palliative   paliative   _____

K. Pronunciation to Spelling

Using the pronunciations that follow, spell the word correctly. Write your response in the space provided.

1. (ah-**GRAFF**-ee-ah) _____

2. (**AN**-yoo-rihzm) _____

3. (kaw-**ZAL**-jee-ah) _____

4. (dis-**FAY**-zee-ah) _____

5. (noo-**RYE**-tis) _____

L. Construct-a-Word

From the following word elements, construct a word that matches the definitions below. Write your response in the space provided.

an-	crani/o	-algesia
quadri-		-esthesia
an-		-tomy
dys-		-phasia
		-plegia

1. without sensitivity to pain _____

2. without feeling or sensation _____

3. a surgical incision into the cranium or skull _____

4. difficult speech _____

5. paralysis of all four extremities and the trunk of the body, caused by injury to the spinal cord at the level of the cervical spine _____

CHAPTER 9

The Blood and Lymphatic Systems

A. Review Checkpoint: Anatomy & Physiology

Completion: Read each statement carefully and write the appropriate answer in the space provided.

1. Red blood cells, tiny biconcave-shaped discs that are thinner in the center than around the edges, are also called _____.

2. Thrombocytes are also known as _____.

3. A stringy, insoluble protein that is the substance of a blood clot is _____.

4. The smallest lymphatic vessels are called _____. (hint: two words)

5. The interstitial fluid picked up by the lymphatic capillaries and eventually returned to the blood is known as _____.

B. Review Checkpoint: Vocabulary

Build-a-Word: Test your word building skills. Using the clues below, build the appropriate medical terms.

1. Build a word that means "stopping or controlling blood."

    _____ + _____ + _____ = _____
    word root   combining vowel   suffix   word

2. Build a word that means "a deficiency in the number of all blood cells."

    _____ + _____ + _____ + _____ = _____
    prefix   word root   combining vowel   suffix   word

3. Build a word that means "a clotting cell."

    _____ + _____ + _____ = _____
    word root   combining vowel   suffix   word

4. Build a word that means "any disease of the lymph glands."

    _____ + _____ + _____ + _____ = _____
    word root   word root   combining vowel   suffix   word

5. Build a word that means "the study of being immune or protected."

    _____ + _____ + _____ = _____
    word root   combining vowel   suffix   word

C. Review Checkpoint: Word Elements

Matching: Match the word elements listed on the left to the appropriate definition on the right.

_____ 1. hyper-   a. unequal

_____ 2. mon/o   b. to clump

_____ 3. agglutin/o   c. excessive

_____ 4. aniso-   d. red, rosy

_____ 5. eosin/o   e. one

D. Review Checkpoint: Pathological Conditions

Completion: Read each statement carefully and write the appropriate answer in the space provided.

1. The type of anemia characterized by the extreme reduction in circulating red blood cells due to their destruction is known as _____ anemia.

2. The type of anemia that results from a deficiency of mature red blood cells and the formation and circulation of megaloblasts with marked shape variation and red blood cell size variation, which is due to a lack of vitamin B_{12}, is known as _____ anemia.

3. A condition in which there is an abnormal increase in the number of red blood cells, granulocytes, and thrombocytes—leading to an increase in blood volume and viscosity (thickness)—is known as _____. (hint: two words)

4. A lymphoid tissue neoplasm that is typically malignant, beginning with a painless enlarged lymph node(s) and progressing to anemia, weakness, intermittent fever, and weight loss, is known as _____.

5. A locally destructive malignant neoplasm of the blood vessels associated with AIDS—typically forming lesions on the skin, visceral organs, or mucous membranes—is known as _____ sarcoma.

E. Review Checkpoint: Diagnostic Techniques, Treatments, and Procedures

Completion: Read each statement carefully and write the appropriate answer in the space provided.

1. An X-ray assessment of the lymphatic system following injection of a contrast medium into the lymph vessels in the hand or foot is known as a(n) _____.

2. The laboratory test that detects the presence of the antibodies to HIV, the virus that causes AIDS, and is used to confirm the validity of ELISA tests is known as the _____ test. (hint: two words)

3. The measurement of the time required for bleeding to stop is known as the _____. (hint: two words)

4. An assessment of red blood cell percentage in the total blood volume is known as the _____.

5. A diagnostic analysis for pernicious anemia is the _____ test.

F. Review Checkpoint: Common Abbreviations

Matching: Match the abbreviation on the left with the correct definition on the right.

_____ 1. Hbg

_____ 2. Ab

_____ 3. PT

_____ 4. ARC

_____ 5. CDC

a. Centers for Disease Control and Prevention

b. AIDS-related complex

c. prothrombin time

d. hemoglobin

e. antibody

G. Review Checkpoint: Putting It All Together

The following questions offer a review of the material studied on the blood and lymphatic systems. Read each question carefully and select or write the most appropriate answer.

1. A substance that can produce a hypersensitive reaction in the body is known as a(n) _____.

2. An abnormal condition of the blood characterized by red blood cells of variable and abnormal size is known as _____.

3. An immature red blood cell is called a(n) _____.

4. A stringy, insoluble protein that is the substance of a blood clot is _____.

5. The scientific study of blood and blood-forming tissues is called _____.

6. An abnormal decrease in the number of white blood cells to fewer than 5,000 per cubic millimeter is known as

   a. thrombocytopenia
   b. erythrocytopenia
   c. agranulocytosis
   d. leukocytopenia

7. An abnormal enlargement of the spleen is known as

   a. splenomegaly
   b. spleenomegaly
   c. splenamegaly
   d. splenomegalie

8. A collection of blood beneath the skin in the form of pinpoint hemorrhages appearing as red-purple discolorations and caused from a decreased number of circulating platelets is known as

   a. polycythemia vera
   b. purpura
   c. multiple myeloma
   d. thalassemia

9. Immunity that is a result of the body developing the ability to defend itself against a specific agent, as a result of having had the disease or from having received an immunization against a disease, is known as

   a. acquired immunity
   b. passive immunity
   c. progressive immunity
   d. natural immunity

10. Immunity with which we are born, also called genetic immunity, is known as

   a. acquired immunity
   b. progressive immunity
   c. passive immunity
   d. natural immunity

11. The body's ability to counteract the effects of pathogens and other harmful agents is known as _____.

12. The masses of lymphatic tissue located in a protective ring, just under the mucous membrane, surrounding the mouth and back of the throat, is known as the _____.

13. A person in a state of having a lack of resistance to pathogens and other harmful agents is said to be _____.

14. Disease-producing microorganisms are known as _____.

15. Cells important to the immune response that mature in the thymus are known as _____.

16. A severe and sometimes fatal hypersensitive (allergic) reaction to a previously encountered antigen is called _____ shock.

17. This benign self-limiting acute infection of the B lymphocytes, usually caused by the Epstein-Barr virus and that affects primarily young adults (15 to 20 years old), is known as

    a. strep throat   c. lymphoma
    b. mononucleosis   d. hypersplenism

18. The most frequent opportunistic infection occurring in persons with AIDS is caused by a common worldwide parasite and is known as

    a. *Pneumocystis carinii* pneumonia   c. systemic lupus erythematosus
    b. sarcoidosis   d. cytomegalovirus

19. The abbreviation *HIV* stands for _____

20. The abbreviation *CDC* stands for _____

H. Labeling

Using the terms listed below, label the following illustration of the lymph ducts and nodes by writing your answers in the spaces provided.

Inguinal nodes

Thoracic duct

Cervical nodes

Submandibular nodes

Axillary nodes

1. _____

2. _____

3. _____

4. _____

5. _____

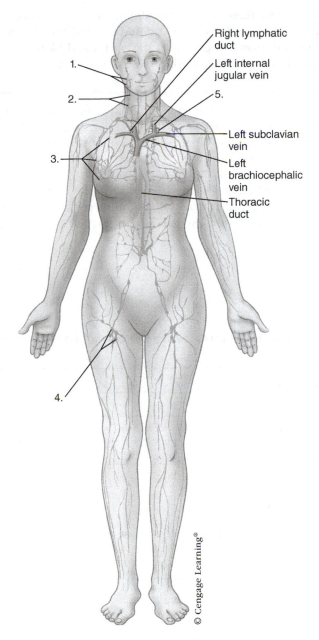

Right lymphatic
duct

Left internal
jugular vein

5.

Left subclavian
vein

Left
brachiocephalic
vein

Thoracic
duct

1.

2.

3.

4.

© Cengage Learning®

Lymphatic ducts and nodes

I. What Is This?

Read the statements that follow and identify the diagnostic technique, treatment, or procedure described. Write the appropriate answer in the space provided.

1. Based on the patient's symptoms, Dr. Smith suspects Mr. Harrill has AIDS. He has ordered a blood test used for screening for an antibody to the AIDS virus. If the outcome is positive, it will indicate probable virus exposure but should be confirmed with another test. What is the abbreviation for this blood test?

   _____

2. The results of the blood test came back positive for Mr. Harrill. Now Dr. Smith is ordering a blood test that detects the presence of the antibodies to HIV and will confirm the validity of the previous test. What is the name of this test? (hint: two words)

   _____

3. Lolita Juarez told her doctor that she feels tired all the time and has no energy. She also has a poor appetite. As part of her examination, Dr. James has ordered a blood test that will measure the concentration of a complex protein-iron compound in the peripheral blood to determine whether or not Lolita is showing signs of anemia. What is the name of this test?

_____

4. Dr. James discovered that Lolita's iron level was low and treated her for a couple of months for iron-deficiency anemia. Lolita has not responded to the treatment, so now Dr. James has ordered a diagnostic analysis for pernicious anemia. What is the name of this test? (hint: two words)

_____

5. George Pollock is suffering from leukemia. During his last visit, the doctor ordered a blood test on George to measure the count of thrombocytes per cubic millimeter of blood and discovered that his thrombocyte level was less than 100,000/mm³, which is indicative of thrombocytopenia. What is the name of this test? (hint: two words)

_____

J. Spelling

Identify the correct spelling of each medical term. Write the correct spelling in the space provided.

1. nutrophil   neutrophil   _____

2. megakarocyte   megakaryocyte   _____

3. hemostasis   hemastasis   _____

4. adnoids   adenoids   _____

5. pathogens   pathagens   _____

K. Pronunciation to Spelling

Using the phonetic pronunciations that follow, spell the word correctly. Write your response in the space provided.

1. (**BAY**-soh-fill) _____

2. (koh-**ag**-yoo-**LAY**-shun) _____

3. (**hee**-mah-**TOL**-oh-jee) _____

4. (**im-YOO**-nih-tee) _____

5. (**LIM**-foh-sight) _____

L. Construct-a-Word

Using the word elements that follow, construct a word that matches the definition provided. Write your response in the space provided.

aniso-	cyt/o	-osis
hyper-	erythr/o	-cyte
pan-	cyt/o	-lysis
	hem/o	-emia
	albumin/o	-penia

1. condition of unequal cell size _____

2. a mature red blood cell _____

3. destruction or breakdown of red blood cells _____

4. an increased level of albumin in the blood _____

5. a marked deficiency in the number of all blood cells _____

The Cardiovascular System

A. Review Checkpoint: Anatomy & Physiology

Completion: Read each statement carefully and write the appropriate answer in the space provided.

1. The heart is the center of the circulatory system. It lies in the middle of the thoracic cavity cradled between the lungs, just behind the sternum, in an area known as the _____.

2. The heart is enclosed by a thin double-walled membranous sac called the _____.

3. The middle, muscular layer of the heart is the _____.

4. Deoxygenated blood enters the _____ from the superior vena cava and the inferior vena cava. (hint: two words)

5. The oxygenated blood is returned to the left atrium of the heart by way of four vessels, two from each lung, known as the _____. (hint: two words)

B. Review Checkpoint: Vocabulary

Build-a-Word: Test your word building skills. Using the clues below, build the appropriate medical terms.

1. Build a word that means "a cell that clots" ("clotting cell").

   _____ + _____ + _____ = _____
   word root   combining vowel   suffix   word

2. Build a word that means "white blood cell."

   _____ + _____ + _____ = _____
   word root   combining vowel   suffix   word

3. Build a word that means "excessive flow of blood."

   _____ + _____ + _____ = _____
   word root   combining vowel   suffix   word

4. Build a word that means "one who specializes in the study of blood."

   _____ + _____ + _____ = _____
   word root   combining vowel   suffix   word

5. Build a word that means "the process of a cell engulfing ('eating') or destroying bacteria."

   _____ + _____ + _____ + _____ = _____
   word root   combining vowel   word root   suffix   word

C. Review Checkpoint: Word Elements

Matching: Match the word elements listed on the left to the appropriate definition on the right.

____ 1. angi/o	a. heart
____ 2. echo-	b. sound
____ 3. megal/o	c. vessel
____ 4. my/o	d. enlarged
____ 5. coron/o	e. muscle

D. Review Checkpoint: Common Signs and Symptoms

Matching: Match the sign or symptom on the left to the appropriate definition on the right.

____ 1. anorexia

____ 2. bradycardia

____ 3. palpitation

____ 4. tachycardia

____ 5. dyspnea

a. difficult breathing

b. abnormal rapidity of heart action, usually defined as a heart rate over 100 beats per minute

c. lack or loss of appetite

d. a slow heart rate characterized by a pulse rate under 60 beats per minute

e. rapid, violent, or throbbing pulsation, as an abnormally rapid throbbing or fluttering of the heart

E. Review Checkpoint: Pathological Conditions

Completion: Read each statement carefully and write the appropriate answer in the space provided.

1. A disease of the heart muscle, primarily affecting the pumping ability of the heart, is known as _____.

2. The narrowing of the arteries that supply the heart muscle, to the extent that adequate blood supply to the myocardium is prevented, is known as _____. (hint: three words)

3. Inflammation of the membrane lining of the valves and chambers of the heart caused by direct invasion of bacteria or other organisms and leading to deformity of the valve cusps is known as _____.

4. A heart attack is also known as a(n) _____. (hint: two words)

5. A localized dilation of an artery formed at a weak point in the vessel wall that balloons out with each pulsation of the artery is known as a(n) _____.

F. Review Checkpoint: Diagnostic Techniques, Treatments, and Procedures

Completion: Read each statement carefully and write the appropriate answer in the space provided.

1. The X-ray visualization of the internal anatomy of the heart and blood vessels after introducing a radiopaque substance that promotes the imaging of internal structures that are otherwise difficult to see on X-ray film is known as a(n) _____.

2. A diagnostic procedure for studying the structure and motion of the heart using ultrasound waves is known as a(n) _____.

3. A graphic record of the electrical action of the heart as reflected from various angles to the surface of the skin is known as a(n) _____.

4. A small, portable monitoring device that makes prolonged electrocardiograph recordings on a portable tape recorder is known as _____ monitoring.

5. A serum _____ test measures the amount of fatty substances (cholesterol, triglycerides, and lipoproteins) in a sample of blood obtained by venipuncture.

G. Review Checkpoint: Common Abbreviations

Matching: Match the abbreviations on the left with the correct definitions on the right.

____	1. CAD	a.	sinoatrial
____	2. DOE	b.	coronary artery disease
____	3. MRI	c.	ventricular fibrillation
____	4. V Fib	d.	magnetic resonance imaging
____	5. SA	e.	dyspnea on exertion

H. Review Checkpoint: Putting It All Together

The following questions offer a review of the material studied on the cardiovascular system. Read each question carefully and select or write the most appropriate answer.

1. Inflammation of the sac-like membrane that covers the heart muscle is known as _____.

2. An arterial condition in which there is thickening, hardening, and loss of elasticity of the walls of arteries—resulting in decreased blood supply—especially to the lower extremities and cerebrum is known as hardening of the arteries or _____.

3. A condition in which the patient has a higher blood pressure than that judged to be normal is known as _____.

4. Enlarged, superficial veins (a twisted dilated vein with incompetent valves) are known as _____ veins.

5. An abnormal circulatory condition characterized by decreased return of venous blood from the legs to the trunk of the body is known as venous _____.

6. A congenital heart disease that is an abnormal opening between the pulmonary artery and the aorta caused by failure of the fetal ductus arteriosis to close after birth is known as

   a. patent ductus arteriosus   c. coarctation of the aorta
   b. tetralogy of Fallot   d. pulmonary stenosis

7. A condition in which the contractions of the atria become extremely rapid, at the rate of between 250 and 350 beats per minute, is known as

   a. atrial fibrillation   c. atrial bradycardia
   b. atrial flutter   d. transposition of the great vessels

8. The extremely rapid, incomplete contractions of the atria resulting in disorganized and uncoordinated twitching of the atria is known as

   a. atrial fibrillation   c. atrial bradycardia
   b. atrial flutter   d. transposition of the great vessels

9. A condition in which the ventricles of the heart beat at a rate greater than 100 beats per minute and characterized by three or more consecutive premature ventricular contractions is known as

   a. ventricular block
   b. ventricular bradycardia

   c. ventricular fibrillation
   d. ventricular tachycardia

10. A form of arteriosclerosis characterized by fatty deposits building up within the inner layers of the walls of large arteries is known as

    a. arteriosclerosis
    b. atherosclerosis

    c. ascites
    d. hepatomegaly

11. Any one of the small flaps on the valves of the heart is known as a(n) _____.

12. The localized or generalized collection of fluid within the body tissues, causing the area to swell, is known as _____.

13. The double-folded membrane that encloses the heart (is "upon" the heart) is known as the _____.

14. Enlargement of the liver is known as _____.

15. Inflammation of the heart muscles is known as _____.

16. The insufficient oxygenation of arterial blood is known as

    a. hypoxemia
    b. anemia

    c. lipidemia
    d. Homan's sign

17. A low-pitched humming or fluttering sound heard on auscultation of the heart is known as a

    a. pacemaker
    b. petechia

    c. murmur
    d. coronary lesion

18. A pounding or racing of the heart associated with normal emotional responses or with heart disorders is known as a

    a. palpitation
    b. rhythm strip

    c. petechia
    d. systole

19. Swelling, usually of the skin of the extremities, that when pressed firmly with a finger will maintain the dent produced by the finger, is known as _____ edema.

    a. palpable
    b. pitting

    c. pulmonary
    d. pericardial

20. The circulation of deoxygenated blood from the right ventricle of the heart to the lungs for oxygenation and back to the left atrium of the heart (from the heart, to the lungs, back to the heart) is known as _____ circulation.

    a. systemic
    b. pericardial

    c. pulmonary
    d. coronary

I. Labeling

Labeling 1

Using the terms listed below, label the following illustration of the linings and layers of the heart in the cardiovascular system by writing your answers in the spaces provided.

Endocardium

Myocardium

Pericardium

Pericardial cavity

Epicardium

1. _____

2. _____

3. _____

4. _____

5. _____

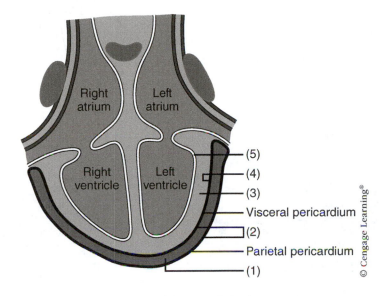

Linings and layers of the heart

Labeling 2

Using the terms listed below, label the following illustrations of pulse points in the body by writing your answers in the spaces provided.

Femoral

Dorsalis pedis

Temporal

Radial

Carotid

Popliteal

Brachial

1. _____

2. _____

3. _____

4. _____

5. _____

6. _____

7. _____

(continued)

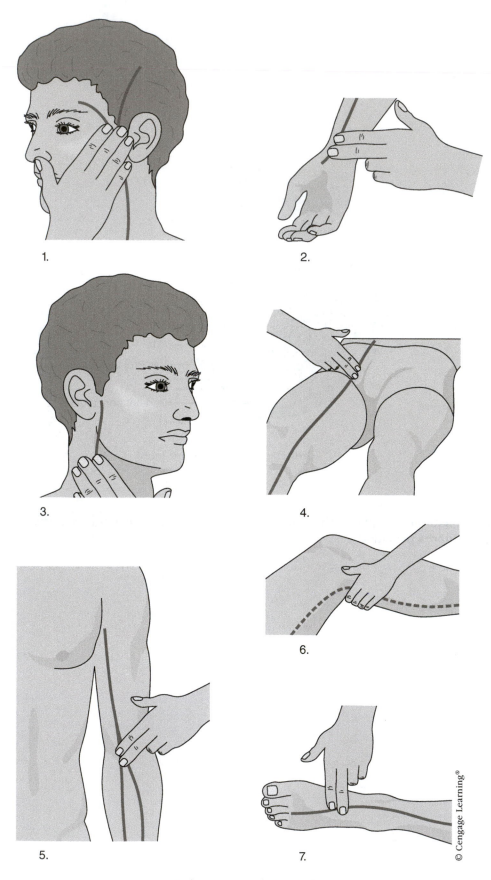

Pulse points of the body

J. What Is This?

Read the statements that follow and identify the diagnostic technique, treatment, or procedure described. Write the appropriate answer in the space provided.

1. Mr. Mason has been experiencing chest pain and discomfort in his left arm. The pain has not intensified but has lingered for a couple of days. He was seen by his internist, who has been treating him for hypertension. After examining Mr. Mason, the physician has ordered a diagnostic procedure in which a catheter will be introduced into a large vein or artery (usually of an arm or a leg) and then is threaded through the circulatory system to the heart. The test should provide detailed information about the structure and function of the heart chambers, valves, and the great vessels. What is the name of this test? (hint: two words)

   _____

2. Mr. Kellar has been complaining of periodic bouts of discomfort in his chest. His physician has ruled out a hiatal hernia and is now planning to run tests to determine if Mr. Kellar has a heart dysrhythmia or evidence of myocardial ischemia. The physician's assistant has placed electrodes on Mr. Kellar's chest, which are attached to a small portable monitoring device that makes prolonged electrocardiograph recordings on a portable tape recorder. Mr. Kellar will wear the apparatus for 24 hours and will conduct normal daily activities. He will return the monitor to the office the next day. What is the name of this test? (hint: two words)

   _____

3. Dr. Benjamin has ordered a test that measures the amount of fatty substances (cholesterol, triglycerides, and lipoproteins) in a sample of blood obtained by venipuncture so he can assess his patient's degree of risk for developing coronary artery disease. What is the name of this blood test? (hint: three words)

   _____

4. Dr. Hart has ordered a diagnostic imaging procedure on her patient to examine his artery to determine the presence of plaque buildup in the artery. The procedure involves the use of a strong magnetic field and radiofrequency waves to produce imaging that is valuable in providing images of the heart, large blood vessels (such as the aorta), brain, and soft tissue. What is the name of this procedure? (hint: three words)

   _____

5. Jessica Smart is being seen by her doctor today for a routine physical examination. One part of the exam consists of a procedure that provides a graphic record (visual representation) of the electrical action of the heart as reflected from various angles to the surface of the skin. What is the name of the record produced by this machine?

   _____

K. Spelling

Identify the correct spelling of each medical term. Write the correct spelling in the space provided.

1. Holter   Halter   _____

2. anomely   anomaly   _____

3. asites   ascites   _____

4. bruit   brewee   _____

5. malaise   malase   _____

L. Pronunciation to Spelling

Using the phonetic pronunciations that follow, spell the word correctly. Write your response in the space provided.

1. (ah-**SIGH**-teez) _____

2. (car-**DYE**-tis) _____

3. (**high**-per-**TEN**-shun) _____

4. (iss-**KEY**-mee-ah) _____

5. (peh-**TEE**-kee-ee) _____

CHAPTER 11

The Respiratory System

A. Review Checkpoint: Anatomy & Physiology

Completion: Read each statement carefully and write the appropriate answer in the space provided.

1. The respiratory system is responsible for the exchange of gases, between the body and the air, a process called _____.

2. The _____ is unique in that it serves as a common passageway for both air and food.

3. The lungs extend from the collarbone to the _____ in the thoracic cavity.

4. During the physical exam, the process of listening for sounds within the body, usually to sounds of thoracic or abdominal viscera, to detect some abnormal condition or to detect fetal heart sounds is known as _____.

5. The use of the fingertips to tap the body lightly but sharply to determine position, size, and consistency of an underlying structure and the presence of fluid or pus in a cavity is known as _____.

B. Review Checkpoint: Vocabulary

Build-a-Word: Test your word building skills. Using the clues below, build the appropriate medical terms.

1. Build a word that means "the double-folded membrane that lines the thoracic cavity."

   _____ + _____ = _____
       word root   suffix   word

2. Build a word that means "pain in the larynx."

   _____ + _____ = _____
       word root   suffix   word

3. Build a word that means "one of the smaller subdivisions of the bronchial tubes."

   _____ + _____ = _____
       word root   suffix   word

4. Build a word that means "inflammation of the nose."

   _____ + _____ = _____
       word root   suffix   word

5. Build a word that means "inflammation of a sinus."

   _____ + _____ = _____
       word root   suffix   word

C. Review Checkpoint: Word Elements

Matching: Match the word elements listed on the left to the appropriate definition on the right.

_____ 1. pector/o   a. bronchus

_____ 2. rhin/o   b. lungs

_____ 3. pne/o   c. chest

_____ 4. pulmon/o   d. nose

_____ 5. bronch/o   e. breathing

D. Review Checkpoint: Common Signs and Symptoms

Matching: Match the sign or symptom on the left to the appropriate definition on the right.

_____ 1. apnea   a. temporary cessation of breathing; "without breathing"

_____ 2. bradypnea   b. nosebleed

_____ 3. dysphonia   c. the act of spitting out saliva or coughing up materials
                                      from the air passageways leading to the lungs

_____ 4. epistaxis

_____ 5. expectoration   d. abnormally slow breathing

                                  e. difficulty speaking; hoarseness

E. Review Checkpoint: Pathological Conditions

Completion: Read each statement carefully and write the appropriate answer in the space provided.

1. Inflammation of the respiratory mucous membranes, known as rhinitis or the common cold, is called _____.

2. Inflammation of the mucous membrane of the bronchial tubes is known as _____.

3. _____ is the presence of pus in a body cavity, especially in the pleural cavity (pyothorax), and is usually the result of a primary infection in the lungs.

4. Inflammation of both the visceral and parietal pleura is known as pleuritis or _____.

5. Another name for black lung disease is coal worker's pneumoconiosis, or _____.

F. Review Checkpoint: Diagnostic Techniques, Treatments, and Procedures

Completion: Read each statement carefully and write the appropriate answer in the space provided.

1. The examination of the interior of the bronchi using a lighted, flexible tube known as a bronchoscope (or endoscope) is known as a(n) _____.

2. The procedure that involves the use of a needle to collect pleural fluid for laboratory analysis or to remove excess pleural fluid or air from the pleural space is known as a(n) _____.

3. A(n) _____ _____ is a specimen of material expectorated from the mouth. If produced after a cough, it may contain (in addition to saliva) material from the throat and bronchi.

4. The visual imaging of the distribution of ventilation or blood flow in the lungs by scanning the lungs after the patient has been injected with or has inhaled radioactive material is known as a(n) _____ _____.

5. The examination of the interior of the larynx using a lighted, flexible tube known as a laryngoscope or endoscope is called a(n) _____.

G. Review Checkpoint: Common Abbreviations

Matching: Match the abbreviations on the left with the correct definitions on the right.

____ 1. CXR   a. upper respiratory infection

____ 2. CDC   b. posteroanterior

____ 3. TST   c. chest X-ray

____ 4. PA   d. Centers for Disease Control and Prevention

____ 5. URI   e. tuberculin skin test

H. Review Checkpoint: Putting It All Together

The following questions offer a review of the material studied on the respiratory system. Read each question carefully and select or write the most appropriate answer.

1. A childhood illness characterized by a barking cough, hoarseness, tachypnea, inspiratory stridor, and laryngeal spasm is known as _____.

2. _____ is an acute upper respiratory infectious disease also known as "whooping cough."

3. Inflammation of the mucous membranes of the nose, usually resulting in obstruction of the nasal passages, rhinorrhea, sneezing, and facial pressure or pain, is known as coryza, or _____.

4. A condition characterized by paroxysmal dyspnea accompanied by wheezing caused by a spasm of the bronchial tubes or by swelling of their mucous membrane is known as _____.

5. A chronic dilation of a bronchus or bronchi, with secondary infection that usually involves the lower portion of the lung, is known as _____.

6. A malignant tumor that originates in the bronchi is

   a. bronchiogenic carcinoma   c. pulmonary adenoma
   b. alveolar carcinoma   d. bronchitis

7. A chronic pulmonary disease characterized by an increase beyond the normal in the size of air spaces distal to the terminal bronchiole, either from dilation of the alveoli or from destruction of their walls, is known as

   a. bronchitis   c. empyema
   b. emphysema   d. hyaline membrane disease

8. A localized collection of pus formed by the destruction of lung tissue and microorganisms by white blood cells that have migrated to the area to fight infection is known as a(n)

   a. pleural effusion   c. lung abscess
   b. empyema   d. pleurisy

9. Inflammation of both the visceral and parietal pleura is known as

   a. pleurisy   c. emphysema
   b. lung abscess   d. pleural effusion

10. Accumulation of fluid in the pleural space, resulting in compression of the underlying portion of the lung, with resultant dyspnea (usually secondary to some other disease) is known as

    a. pleurisy
    b. lung abscess
    c. emphysema
    d. pleural effusion

11. Pus in a body cavity, especially in the pleural cavity, usually the result of a primary infection in the lungs, is known as _____.

12. The accumulation of carbon deposits in the lungs due to breathing smoke or coal dust is known as _____.

13. A lung disease resulting from inhalation of silica (quartz) dust, characterized by formation of small nodules, is known as _____.

14. A lung disease resulting from inhalation of asbestos particles is known as _____.

15. A lung disease resulting from inhalation of cotton, flax, and hemp—also known as brown lung disease—is _____.

16. Lymphatic tissue forming a prominence on the wall of the recess of the nasopharynx is known as

    a. adenoids
    b. bronchi
    c. glottis
    d. bronchioles

17. The sound-producing apparatus of the larynx consisting of the two vocal folds and the intervening space (the epiglottis protects this opening) is known as the

    a. diaphragm
    b. glottis
    c. larynx
    d. oropharynx

18. The external nostrils are known as the

    a. nares
    b. nasopharynx
    c. alveoli
    d. cilia

19. The substance coughed up from the lungs, bronchi, and trachea that is expelled through the mouth is known as

    a. septum
    b. sputum
    c. saliva
    d. empyema

20. A forceful and sometimes violent expiratory effort preceded by a preliminary inspiration is known as

    a. dyspnea
    b. hemoptysis
    c. cough
    d. epistaxis

I. Labeling

Using the terms listed below, label the following illustration of the pathway of air from nose to alveoli by writing your answers in the spaces provided.

Nasal cavity

Epiglottis

Larynx

Trachea

Bronchi

1. _____

2. _____

3. _____

4. _____

5. _____

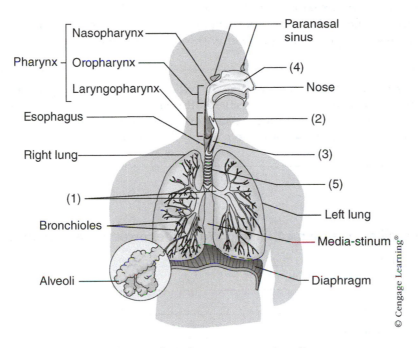

Pathway of air from nose to alveoli

J. What Is This?

Read the statements that follow and identify the diagnostic technique, treatment, or procedure described. Write the appropriate answer in the space provided.

1. Mr. Smoke has had a persistent cough and hoarseness for several months. The doctor has scheduled Mr. Smoke for an examination of the interior of the bronchi using a lighted, flexible tube known as an endoscope in order to observe the air passages for signs of disease and to obtain a biopsy of bronchial tissue for examination. What is the name of this procedure?

_____

2. The physician suspects that Mrs. Cone may have tuberculosis. He has ordered several tests. The medical assistant instructs Mrs. Cone on the first procedure. She tells Mrs. Cone that the specimen should be collected preferably in the morning before eating or drinking. She encourages Mrs. Cone to cough deeply (from as far down as possible) and to place the material expectorated from the mouth in the labeled container. The medical assistant also instructs Mrs. Cone to place the first container in the labeled bag and return it to the office laboratory the same day. What is the name of this test? (hint: two words)

_____

3. Once the medical assistant is sure that Mrs. Cone understands the process of correctly collecting the specimen, she prepares to administer an injection of PPD intradermally. This test is used to determine past or present tuberculosis infection present in the body. Upon administration of the medication, the medical assistant instructs Mrs. Cone to return to the office in 48 hours to have the results recorded. What is the name of this test? (hint: three words)

_____

4. When Mrs. Cone returned to the office to learn the results of the PPD injection, the result was positive and indicated the need for further testing. The doctor ordered the use of high-energy electromagnetic waves passing through the body onto a photographic film to produce a picture of the lungs for diagnosis and therapy. What is the name of this procedure? (hint: two words)

_____

5. Mr. Brown has worked in a textile mill for over 20 years. His physician suspects that he may be suffering from byssinosis (brown lung disease). Mr. Brown's complaint is continued wheezing and tightness in the chest, resulting in dyspnea. The doctor has ordered a series of tests to assess Mr. Brown's respiratory function. What is the name of these tests? (hint: three words)

_____

K. Spelling

Identify the correct spelling of each medical term. Write the correct spelling in the space provided.

1. larynx   larnyx   _____

2. pleura   plura   _____

3. dyspnea   dysnea   _____

4. hemoptosis   hemoptysis   _____

5. croop   croup   _____

L. Pronunciation to Spelling

Using the phonetic pronunciations that follow, spell the word correctly. Write your response in the space provided.

1. (**AY**-peks) _____

2. (**BRONG**-kigh) _____

3. (**LAIR**-inks) _____

4. (diss-**FOH**-nee-ah) _____

5. (ep-ih-**STAKS**-is) _____

CHAPTER 12

The Digestive System

A. Review Checkpoint: Anatomy & Physiology

Completion: Read each statement carefully and write the appropriate answer in the space provided.

1. The first part of the digestive tract is the _____ cavity.

2. The _____ forms the anterior, upper roof of the mouth and is supported by bone. It has irregular ridges or folds in its mucous membrane lining. (hint: two words)

3. During the process of chewing food, the tongue aids the digestive process by moving the food around to mix it with saliva, shaping it into a ball-like mass called a(n) _____.

4. The digestive enzyme contained in saliva that aids in the digestion of carbohydrates is _____.

5. The _____ regulates the passage of food from the stomach into the duodenum. (hint: two words)

B. Review Checkpoint: Vocabulary

Build-a-Word: Test your word building skills. Using the clues below, build the appropriate medical terms.

1. Build a word that literally means "without eating" (a condition characterized by the loss of ability to swallow).

   _____ + _____ = _____
   without   to eat   complete word

2. Build a word that literally means "difficult or bad digestion" (a vague feeling of epigastric discomfort after eating).

   _____ + _____ = _____
   bad, difficult   digestion   complete word

3. Build a word that means "surgical removal of the appendix."

   _____ + _____ = _____
   appendix   surgical removal   complete word

4. Build a word that means "inflammation of the tongue."

   _____ + _____ = _____
   tongue   inflammation   complete word

5. Build a word that literally means a "fat enzyme" (an enzyme that aids in the digestion of fats).

   _____ + _____ = _____
   fat   enzyme   complete word

C. Review Checkpoint: Word Elements

Matching: Match the word elements listed on the left to the appropriate definition on the right.

_____ 1. choledoch/o

_____ 2. cheil/o

_____ 3. lapar/o

_____ 4. -emesis

_____ 5. -phagia

a. to vomit

b. to eat

c. common bile duct

d. abdominal wall

e. lips

D. Review Checkpoint: Common Signs and Symptoms

Matching: Match the sign or symptom on the left to the appropriate definition on the right.

_____ 1. borborygmus

_____ 2. diarrhea

_____ 3. emaciation

_____ 4. eructation

_____ 5. melena

a. excessive leanness caused by disease or lack of nutrition

b. an abnormal, black, tarry stool containing digested blood

c. an audible abdominal sound produced by hyperactive intestinal peristalsis

d. the frequent passage of loose, watery stools

e. the act of bringing up air from the stomach with a characteristic sound through the mouth; belching

E. Review Checkpoint: Pathological Conditions

Completion: Read each statement carefully and write the appropriate answer in the space provided.

1. Decreased mobility of the lower two-thirds of the esophagus along with constriction of the lower esophageal sphincter is known as _____.

2. Small inflammatory noninfectious ulcerated lesions occurring on the lips, tongue, and inside the cheeks of the mouth; also called canker sores; are known as _____. (hint: two words)

3. Inflammation of the vermiform appendix is known as _____.

4. Swollen, twisted (tortuous) veins located in the distal end of the esophagus are known as _____. (hint: two words)

5. An unnaturally distended or swollen vein (called a varicosity) in the distal rectum or anus is known as a(n) _____.

F. Review Checkpoint: Diagnostic Techniques, Treatments, and Procedures

Completion: Read each statement carefully and write the appropriate answer in the space provided.

1. The surgical removal of an inflamed appendix is known as a(n) _____.

2. The infusion of a radiopaque contrast medium, barium sulfate, into the rectum and held in the lower intestinal tract while X-ray films are obtained of the lower GI tract is known as a lower GI series or a(n) _____. (hint: two words)

3. The surgical removal of the gallbladder is known as a(n) _____.

4. The process of viewing the entire length of the small intestine using an ingestible video camera with a light source, which is enclosed in a capsule (about the size of a large vitamin pill), is known as a(n) _____. (hint: two words)

5. The analysis of a stool sample to determine the presence of blood not visible to the naked eye is known as a stool analysis for _____. (hint: two words)

G. Review Checkpoint: Common Abbreviations

Matching: Match the abbreviations on the left with the correct definitions on the right.

_____	1. Ba	a. lower esophageal sphincter
_____	2. LES	b. nausea and vomiting
_____	3. N&V	c. small bowel series
_____	4. SBS	d. barium
_____	5. TPN	e. total parenteral nutrition

H. Review Checkpoint: Putting It All Together

The following questions offer a review of the material studied on the digestive system. Read each question carefully and select, or write, the most appropriate answer.

1. The anterior, upper roof of the mouth that has irregular ridges or folds in its mucous membrane lining is known as the _____. (hint: two words)

2. The sphincter that regulates the passage of food from the stomach into the duodenum is known as the _____ sphincter.

3. The yellowish-green secretion of the liver that breaks apart fats, preparing them for further digestion and absorption, is known as _____.

4. Another name for the digestive tract is the gastrointestinal tract or the _____. (hint: two words)

5. The sphincter in the stomach that controls passage of food from the esophagus into the stomach is known as the lower esophageal sphincter or the _____ sphincter.

6. Decreased motility of the esophagus is known as

   a. aphthous stomatitis
   b. gastroesophageal reflux
   c. achalasia
   d. celiac disease

7. Telescoping of a portion of proximal intestine into distal intestine, usually in the ileocecal region (causing an obstruction), is known as

   a. volvulus
   b. intussusception
   c. Hirschsprung's disease
   d. irritable bowel syndrome

8. A digestive tract inflammation of a chronic nature causing fever, cramping, diarrhea, weight loss, and anorexia is known as

   a. Crohn's disease
   b. Hirschsprung's disease
   c. ileus
   d. celiac disease

9. Another name for canker sores is

   a. aphthous stomatitis
   b. icterus
   c. dyspepsia
   d. oral leukoplakia

10. Tooth decay is also known as

    a. dysentery
    b. dental caries

    c. periodontal disease
    d. oral leukoplakia

11. The insertion of a needle or trochar into the abdominal cavity to remove excess fluid (with the person in a sitting position) is known as a paracentesis or _____.

12. The use of very high-frequency sound waves to provide visualization of the internal organs of the body cavity that contains the liver, gallbladder, bile ducts, pancreas, kidneys, bladder, and ureters is known as a(n) _____ ultrasound.

13. A lower GI series is also known as a(n) _____. (hint: two words)

14. The surgical removal of the gallbladder is known as a(n) _____.

15. A procedure used to measure and monitor the amount of gastric acid reflux into the esophagus during a two-day period of time, in which the patient has a small capsule containing a radiotransmitter attached to the wall of the esophagus, is known as a(n) _____ study.

16. Which of the following medical terms means "greater than normal amounts of fat in the feces, characterized by frothy foul-smelling fecal matter that floats"?

    a. steatorrhea
    b. dentin

    c. chime
    d. bolus

17. Which of the following medical terms means "abnormal presence of gallstones in the gallbladder," "abnormal condition of gallstones"?

    a. cholecystitis
    b. cholelithiasis

    c. hepatitis
    d. glycogenolysis

18. Which of the following terms means "pertaining to the stomach and the esophagus"?

    a. gastrointestinal
    b. reflux

    c. gastroesophageal
    d. peritoneal

19. Which of the following terms means "inflammation of the gums"?

    a. gingivitis
    b. esophagitis

    c. hepatitis
    d. pharyngitis

20. Which of the following terms means "vomiting of blood"?

    a. hemoptysis
    b. hematemesis

    c. hemorrhage
    d. Hemoccult

I. Labeling

Labeling 1

Using the terms listed below, label the following illustration of the accessory organs of the digestive system by writing your answers in the spaces provided.

Common bile duct

Cystic duct

Gallbladder

Liver

Pancreas

1. _____

2. _____

3. _____

4. _____

5. _____

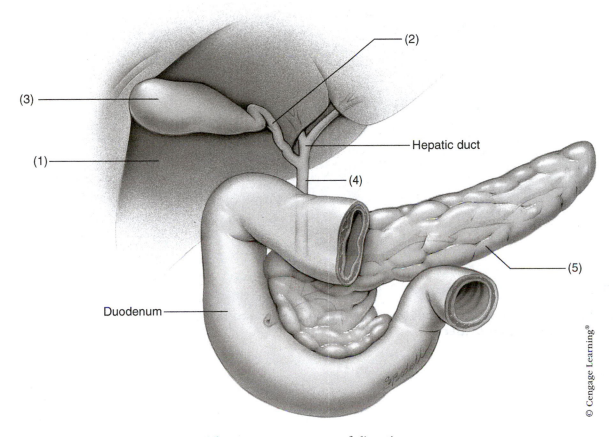

The accessory organs of digestion

Labeling 2

Using the terms listed below, label the following illustration of the stomach by writing your answers in the spaces provided.

Rugae

Pylorus

Fundus

Body

Pyloric sphincter

1. _____

2. _____

3. _____

4. _____

5. _____

(continued)

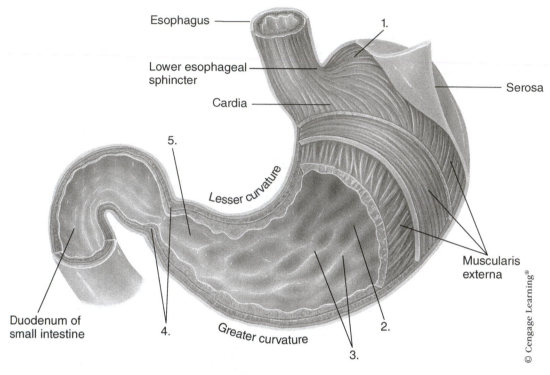

Esophagus

Lower esophageal sphincter

Cardia

1.

Serosa

5.

Lesser curvature

Duodenum of small intestine

4.

Greater curvature

2.

3.

Muscularis externa

© Cengage Learning®

The Stomach

Labeling 3

Using the terms listed below, label the following illustration of the layers of the tooth by writing your answers in the spaces provided.

Neck

Enamel

Root

Dentin

Crown

1. _____

2. _____

3. _____

4. _____

5. _____

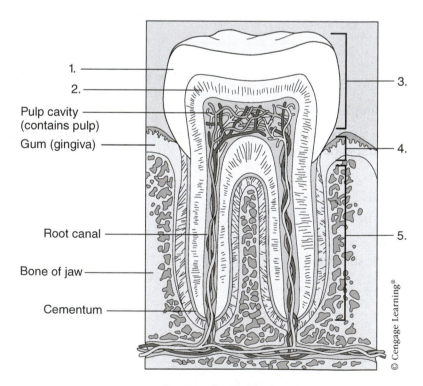

1.

2.

Pulp cavity (contains pulp)

Gum (gingiva)

3.

4.

Root canal

5.

Bone of jaw

Cementum

© Cengage Learning®

Layers of a tooth

J. What Is This?

Read the statements that follow and identify the diagnostic technique, treatment, or procedure described. Write the appropriate answer in the space provided.

1. Dr. Hughes has ordered a procedure for Ms. Smith to remove a large amount of ascitic fluid from her distended abdomen. This procedure will reduce pressure and should help her breathe more effectively. Ms. Smith will be placed in a sitting position and a large needle or trochar will be inserted into the abdominal cavity to remove the excess fluid. What procedure is this? (hint: two possible choices)

   _____

2. William Gaskin is scheduled for a procedure tomorrow at the Diagnostic Center. He will receive an infusion of a radiopaque contrast medium, barium sulfate, into the rectum. The contrast medium will remain in the lower intestinal tract while X-ray films are obtained of the lower GI tract. What procedure is this? (hint: two possible choices)

   _____

3. Juan Pedros has been referred to the outpatient clinic by Dr. Jones. The doctor suspects that Juan may have colonic polyps, based on his symptoms. This procedure involves the direct visualization of the lining of the large intestine using a fiberoptic colonoscope. What procedure is this?

   _____

4. Allyson Blue was admitted to the emergency department at the local hospital with a diagnosis of overdose of sleeping pills. The physician on duty has ordered the irrigation, or washing out, of Allyson's stomach with sterile water or a saline solution in order to remove the toxic substances from her stomach. What procedure is this? (hint: two words)

   _____

5. Mark Davis had surgery today for the surgical repair of a hernia, in which the defect was closed using sutures, mesh, or wire. When Mark is discharged, he will be on activity restriction with no heavy labor or lifting for at least three weeks following surgery. What surgery is this?

   _____

K. Spelling

Identify the correct spelling of each medical term. Write the correct spelling in the space provided.

1. ascitic fluid   asidic fluid   _____

2. spincter   sphincter   _____

3. chyme   khyme   _____

4. peristalsus   peristalsis   _____

5. pharynx   pharanyx   _____

L. Pronunciation to Spelling

Using the phonetic pronunciations that follow, spell the word correctly. Write your response in the space provided.

1. (dye-**JEST**-shun) _____

2. (eh-**MULL**-sih-figh) _____

3. (gah-**VAZH**) _____

4. (**GLIGH**-koh-jen) _____

5. (**SFINGK**-ter) _____

CHAPTER 13

The Endocrine System

A. Review Checkpoint: Anatomy & Physiology

Completion: Read each statement carefully and write the appropriate answer in the space provided.

1. Another name for the neurohypophysis is the ———————— pituitary gland.

2. The ———————— gland controls metabolism in the body.

3. Insulin is secreted by the ————————.

4. The female sex glands, also known as the female gonads, are the ————————.

5. The male gonads, or testicles, are also known as the ————————.

B. Review Checkpoint: Vocabulary

Build-a-Word: Test your word-building skills. Using the clues below, build the appropriate medical terms.

1. Build a word that means "enlargement of the extremities."

   ————————— + ————————— + ————————— = —————————
      word root   vowel   suffix   word

2. Build a word that means "any disease of a gland, characterized by enlargement."

   ————————— + ————————— + ————————— = —————————
      word root   combining vowel   suffix   word

3. Build a word that means "a physician who specializes in the medical practice of treating the diseases and disorders of the endocrine system."

   ————————— + ————————— + ————————— + ————————— = —————————
      prefix   word root   combining vowel   suffix   word

4. Build a word that means "the formation or production of glycogen from fatty acids and proteins instead of carbohydrates."

   ————————— + ————————— + ————————— = —————————
      word root   combining vowel   suffix   word

5. Build a word that means "elevated blood sugar level," "excessive blood sugar."

   ————————— + ————————— + ————————— = —————————
      prefix   word root   suffix   word

C. Review Checkpoint: Word Elements

Matching: Match the word elements listed on the left to the appropriate definition on the right.

_____ 1. aden/o   a. poisons

_____ 2. crin/o   b. sugar, sweet

_____ 3. glyc/o   c. gland

_____ 4. oxy-   d. secrete

_____ 5. toxic/o   e. sharp, quick

D. Review Checkpoint: Pathological Conditions

Completion: Read each statement carefully and write the appropriate answer in the space provided.

1. A chronic metabolic condition characterized by the gradual noticeable enlargement and elongation of the bones of the face, jaw, and extremities due to hypersecretion of the human growth hormone after puberty is known as _____.

2. A condition caused by a deficiency in the secretion of antidiuretic hormone (ADH) by the posterior pituitary gland, characterized by large amounts of urine and sodium excreted from the body, is known as _____. (hint: two words)

3. A proportional overgrowth of the body's tissue due to the hypersecretion of the human growth hormone before puberty is known as _____.

4. Hyperplasia of the thyroid gland is known as a(n) _____.

5. Graves' disease is also known as _____.

E. Review Checkpoint: Diagnostic Techniques, Treatments, and Procedures

Completion: Read each statement carefully and write the appropriate answer in the space provided.

1. A blood glucose sample taken usually early in the morning after the person has been without food or drink since midnight is called a(n) _____ test. (hint: three words)

2. A test that evaluates a person's ability to tolerate a concentrated oral glucose load by measuring the glucose levels is known as a(n) _____ test. (hint: two words)

3. A blood test that shows the average level of glucose in an individual's blood during the last 3 months is known as a(n) _____ test. (hint: two words)

4. Tests that measure the blood levels of the hormones T3, T4, and TSH are known as thyroid _____ tests.

5. An examination that determines the position, size, shape, and physiological function of the thyroid gland through the use of radionuclear scanning is known as a(n) _____. (hint: two words)

F. Review Checkpoint: Common Abbreviations

Matching: Match the abbreviations on the left with the correct definitions on the right.

_____ 1. ADH   a. potassium

_____ 2. HDL   b. antidiuretic hormone

_____ 3. Na   c. radioactive iodine uptake

_____ 4. K   d. sodium

_____ 5. RAI   e. high-density lipoprotein

G. Review Checkpoint: Putting It All Together

The following questions offer a review of the material studied on the endocrine system. Read each question carefully and select, or write, the most appropriate answer.

1. Inflammation of the thyroid gland is known as _____.

2. An acute, sometimes fatal, incident of overactivity of the thyroid gland resulting in excessive secretion of thyroid hormone is known as _____. (hint: two words)

3. A life-threatening disease process due to failure of the adrenal cortex to secrete mineralocorticoids and glucocorticoids, characterized by low blood glucose, low blood sodium, weight loss, and increased pigmentation of the skin, is known as _____ disease.

4. A condition of the adrenal gland in which a cluster of symptoms occurs as a result of an excessive amount of cortisol circulating in the blood, characterized by central obesity, round "moon" face, and a buffalo hump, is known as _____ syndrome.

5. Development of male secondary sex characteristics in the female due to the excessive secretion of adrenocortical androgens from the adrenal cortex is known as _____.

6. Which of the following identifies a disorder of the blood vessels of the retina of the eye, in which the capillaries of the retina experience localized areas of microaneurysms, hemorrhages, leakage, and scarring?

   a. gestational diabetes
   b. diabetic retinopathy
   c. diabetes insipidus
   d. diabetic neuropathy

7. An acute or chronic destructive inflammatory condition of the pancreas is known as

   a. hepatitis
   b. pancreatic cancer
   c. pancreatitis
   d. cholecystitis

8. A chronic metabolic condition characterized by gradual, noticeable enlargement and elongation of the bones of the face, jaw, and extremities due to oversecretion of the pituitary gland after puberty is known as

   a. acromegaly
   b. gigantism
   c. dwarfism
   d. hypothyroidism

9. A condition in which there is an abnormal underdevelopment of the body—characterized by extremely short height and usually caused by an undersecretion of the pituitary gland before puberty—is known as

   a. acromegaly
   b. gigantism
   c. dwarfism
   d. hyperthyroidism

10. Which of the following terms means a metabolic disorder of the pituitary gland due to a deficiency in secretion of the antidiuretic hormone, characterized by extreme polydipsia and polyuria?

    a. gestational diabetes
    b. diabetic retinopathy
    c. diabetes insipidus
    d. diabetic neuropathy

11. A physician who specializes in the medical practice of treating diseases and disorders of the endocrine system is called a(n) _____.

12. A hormone produced by the adrenal medulla that plays an important role in the body's response to stress by increasing the heart rate, dilating the bronchioles, and releasing glucose into the bloodstream is _____.

13. _____ is an abnormal condition characterized by a marked outward protrusion of the eyeballs.

14. An excessive amount of insulin in the body is known as _____.

15. An elevated blood sodium level is called _____.

16. Which of the following terms describes a less than normal blood calcium level?

    a. hypocalcemia
    b. hypoglycemia
    c. hyponatremia
    d. hypokalemia

17. Which of the following terms describes a less than normal blood potassium level?

    a. hypocalcemia
    b. hypoglycemia
    c. hyponatremia
    d. hypokalemia

18. Which of the following terms means "excessive thirst"?

    a. polydipsia
    b. polyphagia
    c. polyphasia
    d. polyuria

19. Which of the following terms means "a group of symptoms occurring together, indicative of a particular disease or abnormality"?

    a. myxedema
    b. tetany
    c. syndrome
    d. gigantism

20. Which of the following terms refers to a condition characterized by severe cramping and twitching of the muscles and sharp flexion of the wrist and ankle joints (a complication of hypocalcemia)?

    a. myxedema
    b. tetany
    c. syndrome
    d. gigantism

H. Labeling

Using the terms listed below, label the following diagram of the glands of the endocrine system by writing your answers in the spaces provided.

Pituitary

Thyroid

Liver

Pancreas

Ovaries

1. _____

2. _____

3. _____

4. _____

5. _____

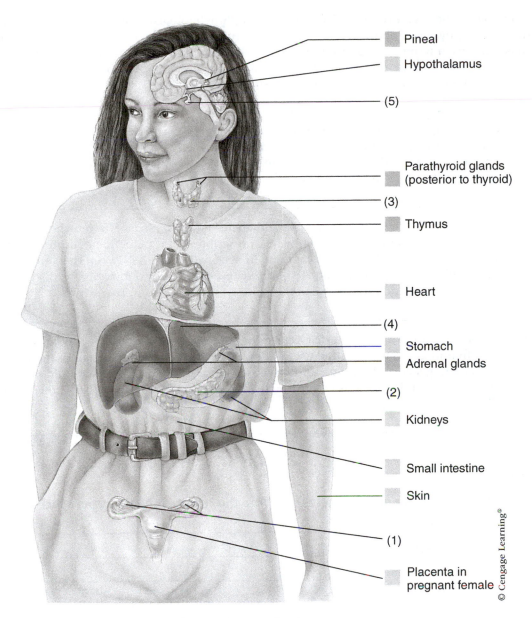

Pineal

Hypothalamus

(5)

Parathyroid glands
(posterior to thyroid)

(3)

Thymus

Heart

(4)

Stomach

Adrenal glands

(2)

Kidneys

Small intestine

Skin

(1)

Placenta in
pregnant female

Glands of the endocrine system

I. What Is This?

Read the statements that follow and identify the diagnostic technique, treatment, or procedure described. Write the appropriate answer in the space provided.

1. Mrs. Jonas was seen by her ophthalmologist today for an eye exam. It has been over four years since Mrs. Jonas has had an eye exam. As the physician examined the interior of Mrs. Jonas's left eye, he noticed some leakage of the vessels in the retina. When questioned, Mrs. Jonas denied any history of diabetes. The doctor ordered a blood test to determine Mrs. Jonas's glucose level at that time. This blood test measured the amount of glucose in the blood at the time the sample was drawn (around 3:45 p.m.). What is the name of this test? (hint: three words)

2. Mrs. Jonas's blood glucose level was 375 mg/dL. The ophthalmologist immediately referred Mrs. Jonas to her primary care physician. She was seen the next morning. The primary care physician requested that Mrs. Jonas not have anything to eat after midnight and come in the next morning for a blood glucose test. This was a sample of blood taken early in the morning after the person has been without food or drink since midnight. What is the name of this test? (hint: three words)

_____

3. Mrs. Jonas's blood sugar level was determined to be 200 mg/dL at the time of her visit with Dr. Smith, her primary care physician. He then ordered an additional blood test that shows the average level of glucose in Mrs. Jonas's blood during the last three months. The normal range for this test is 4%–5.9%. What is the name of this test? (hint: two words)

_____

4. All of the tests confirmed the diagnosis of type II diabetes for Mrs. Jonas. She returned to Dr. Smith for instructions on an appropriate diet plan for her, prescriptions for diabetic medications, and a complete physical exam since she had not had one in over two years. As Dr. Smith examined Mrs. Jonas, he noticed a nodule on her thyroid gland. He ordered an ultrasound examination to distinguish solid thyroid nodules from cystic nodules. What is the name of this test? (hint: two words)

_____

5. Dr. Smith also ordered an examination that determines the position, size, shape, and physiological function of the thyroid gland through the use of radionuclear scanning. An image of the thyroid gland is recorded and visualized after a radioactive substance is given. This test would be helpful in diagnosing the nodules in the neck as either functioning or nonfunctioning. What is the name of this test? (hint: two words)

_____

J. Spelling

Identify the correct spelling of each medical term. Write the correct spelling in the space provided.

1. euthyroid   euthroid   _____

2. exophthalmia   exopthalmia   _____

3. tetney   tetany   _____

4. syndrome   syndrohm   _____

5. acramegaly   acromegaly   _____

K. Pronunciation to Spelling

Using the phonetic pronunciations that follow, spell the word correctly. Write your response in the space provided.

1. (**ad**-eh-**NOP**-ah-thee) _____

2. (**KREE**-tin-izm) _____

3. (yoo-**THIGH**-royd) _____

4. (**eck**-sof-**THAL**-mee-ah) _____

5. (**high**-poff-ih-**SEK**-toh-mee) _____

L. Construct-a-Word

Using the word elements that follow, construct words that match the definitions below. Be sure to drop the combining vowel when necessary. Write your response in the space provided.

endo-	crin/o	-ia
poly-	calc/o	-logist
ex-	ophthalm/o	-uria
hyper-	glycos/o	-emia
		-dipsia

1. a physician who specializes in the medical practice of treating the diseases and disorders of the endocrine system _____

2. an abnormal condition characterized by a marked outward protrusion of the eyeballs _____

3. the presence of sugar in the urine _____

4. elevated blood calcium level _____

5. excessive thirst _____

CHAPTER 14

The Special Senses

A. Review Checkpoint: Anatomy & Physiology

Completion: Read each statement carefully and write the appropriate answer in the space provided.

1. The _____ is the tough, fibrous membrane that maintains the shape of the eyeball and serves as a protective covering for the eye; the white portion of the eye.

2. The _____ is a thin mucous membrane layer that lines the anterior part of the eye, which is exposed to air, and the inner part of the eyelids.

3. The _____ controls the amount of light entering the eye by contracting or dilating.

4. The bending of light rays as they pass through the various structures of the eye to produce a clear image on the retina is known as _____.

5. The tube leading from the auricle to the middle ear is called the _____. (hint: three words)

B. Review Checkpoint: Vocabulary

Build-a-Word: Test your word-building skills. Using the clues below, build the appropriate medical terms.

1. Build a word that means "inflammation of the mastoid process."

   _____ + _____ = _____

      word root   suffix   word

2. Build a word that means "a recording of the faintest sounds an individual is able to hear."

   _____ + _____ + _____ = _____

      word root   combining vowel   suffix   word

3. Build a word that means "drainage from the ear."

   _____ + _____ + _____ = _____

      word root   combining vowel   suffix   word

4. Build a word that means "drooping of the upper eyelid."

   _____ + _____ + _____ = _____

      word root   combining vowel   suffix   word

5. Build a word that means "flow of tears."

   _____ + _____ + _____ = _____

      word root   combining vowel   suffix   word

C. Review Checkpoint: Word Elements

Matching: Match the word elements listed on the left to the appropriate definition on the right.

_____ 1. ambi-   a. eardrum

_____ 2. ambly/o   b. ear

_____ 3. glauc/o   c. gray, silver

_____ 4. ot/o   d. both, both sides

_____ 5. tympan/o   e. dull

D. Review Checkpoint: Pathological Conditions

Completion: Read each statement carefully and write the appropriate answer in the space provided.

1. When the lens of the eye becomes progressively cloudy, losing its normal transparency and thus altering the perception of images due to the interference of light transmission to the retina, the patient is said to have a(n) _____.

2. A "turning out" or eversion of the eyelash margins (especially the lower eyelid) from the eyeball, leading to exposure of the eyelid and eyeball surface and lining, is known as a(n) _____.

3. A bacterial infection of an eyelash follicle or sebaceous gland originating with redness, swelling, and mild tenderness in the margin of the eyelash is known as a hordeolum, or _____.

4. Hearing loss caused by the breakdown of the transmission of sound waves through the middle and/or external ear is known as _____ deafness.

5. The medical term for inflammation of the outer or external ear canal, also known as "swimmer's ear," is _____. (hint: two words)

E. Review Checkpoint: Diagnostic Techniques, Treatments, and Procedures

Completion: Read each statement carefully and write the appropriate answer in the space provided.

1. The process of measuring how well an individual hears various frequencies of sound waves is known as _____.

2. An examination, known as the tuning fork test, compares bone conduction and air conduction as the base of a vibrating tuning fork is placed on the person's mastoid bone and held there until sound can no longer be heard, at which time it is quickly moved in front of the ear near the ear canal. At this time, it is determined if the person continues to hear the sound at the ear canal. The tuning fork test is also known as the _____ test.

3. A surgical procedure with insertion of a small ventilation tube introduced into the inferior segment of the tympanic membrane is known as a tympanotomy or a(n) _____.

4. Extraction of a small segment of the iris to open an anterior chamber angle and permit the flow of aqueous humor between the anterior and posterior chambers, thus relieving intraocular pressure, is known as a(n) _____.

5. The measurement of the thickness of the cornea is known as _____.

F. Review Checkpoint: Common Abbreviations

Matching: Match the abbreviations on the left with the correct definitions on the right.

____ 1. ECCE a. visual acuity

____ 2. IOP b. extracapsular cataract extraction

____ 3. PEARL c. intraocular pressure

____ 4. VA d. extraocular movement

____ 5. EOM e. pupils equal and reactive to light

G. Review Checkpoint: Putting It All Together

The following questions offer a review of the material studied in the special senses chapter. Read each question carefully and select, or write, the most appropriate answer.

1. A refractive error in which the lens of the eye cannot focus on an image accurately, resulting in impaired close vision that is blurred due to the light rays focused behind the retina because the eyeball is shorter than normal, is known as farsightedness or _____.

2. A refractive error in which the lens of the eye cannot focus on an image accurately, resulting in impaired distance vision that is blurred due to the light rays focused in front of the retina because the eyeball is longer than normal, is known as nearsightedness or _____.

3. A refractive error occurring after the age of 40, when the lens of the eye(s) cannot focus on an image accurately due to its decreasing loss of elasticity, is known as _____.

4. An irregular growth developing as a fold in the conjunctiva, usually on the nasal side of the cornea, that can disrupt vision if it extends over the pupil is known as a(n) _____.

5. Convergent strabismus (cross-eye) is also known as _____.

6. An infection or inflammation of the labyrinth or the inner ear—specifically the three semicircular canals in the inner ear, which are fluid-filled chambers and control balance—is known as

   a. labyrinthitis
   b. impacted cerumen
   c. mastoiditis
   d. keratitis

7. A chronic inner ear disease in which there is an overaccumulation of endolymph characterized by recurring episodes of vertigo, hearing loss, feeling of pressure or fullness in the affected ear, and tinnitus is known as

   a. mastoiditis
   b. Ménière's disease
   c. conductive deafness
   d. suppurative otitis media

8. Which of the following terms refers to a middle ear infection?

   a. otitis media
   b. otosclerosis
   c. otitis externa
   d. labyrinthitis

9. Which of the following terms refers to a purulent collection of fluid in the middle ear causing the person to experience pain, an elevation of temperature, dizziness, decreased hearing, vertigo, and tinnitus?

   a. otitis exterma
   b. serous otitis media
   c. suppurative otitis media
   d. labyrinthitis

10. Which of the following terms refers to a collection of clear fluid in the middle ear that may follow acute otitis media or be due to an obstruction of the eustachian tube?

    a. otitis externa
    b. serous otitis media
    c. suppurative otitis media
    d. labyrinthitis

11. A surgical repair of the eardrum with a tissue graft is known as a myringoplasty or a(n) _____.

12. Loss of hearing due to the natural aging process is known as _____.

13. _____ is a medical term that means "containing pus."

14. A(n) _____ is an instrument used to examine the nasopharynx and the eustachian tube.

15. _____ is a sensation of spinning around or of having things in the room or area spinning around the person; a result of disturbance of the equilibrium.

16. Which of the following terms means "inversion, turning inward, of the edge of the eyelid"?

    a. ectropion
    b. entropion
    c. esotropia
    d. exotropia

17. Which of the following terms means "inflammation of the lacrimal gland"?

    a. cycloplegia
    b. conjunctivitis
    c. dacryoadenitis
    d. dacryorrhea

18. Which of the following terms means "loss of vision, or blindness, in one-half of the visual field"?

    a. iridocyclitis
    b. hemianopsia
    c. exotropia
    d. keratoconus

19. Which of the following terms means "the examination of the fundus of the eye, the base or the deepest part of the eye, with an instrument called an ophthalmoscope"?

    a. fundoscopy
    b. otoscopy
    c. nystagmus
    d. phacoemulcification

20. Which of the following terms means "involuntary, rhythmic jerking movements of the eye—movements that can be from side to side, up and down, or a combination of both"?

    a. keratomycosis
    b. presbyopia
    c. nystagmus
    d. uveitis

H. Labeling

Labeling 1

Using the terms listed below, label the following illustration of the structures of the ear by writing your answers in the spaces provided.

Auricle

Eustachian tube

Tympanic membrane

Semicircular canals

Stapes

1. _____

2. _____

3. _____

4. _____

5. _____

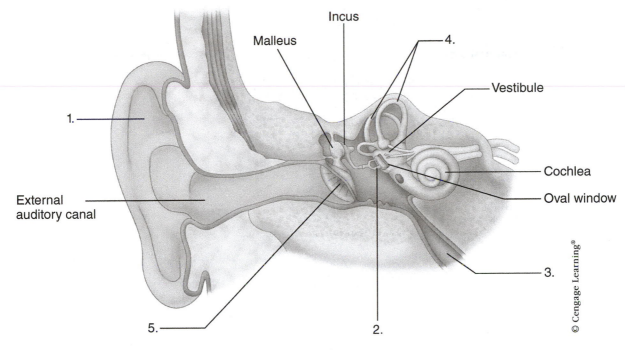

Incus

Malleus

4.

Vestibule

1.

External
auditory canal

Cochlea

Oval window

3.

5.

2.

© Cengage Learning®

Structures of the ear

Labeling 2

Using the terms listed below, label the following illustration of the front view of the eye by writing your answers in the spaces provided.

Inner canthus

Iris

Conjunctiva

Pupil

Sclera

1. _____

2. _____

3. _____

4. _____

5. _____

(continued)

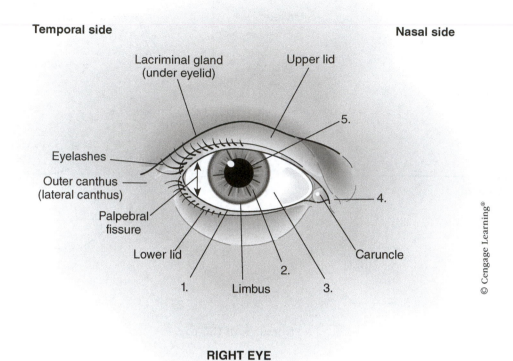

RIGHT EYE

Front view of the eye

Labeling 3

Using the terms listed below, label the following illustration of the structures of the eye by writing your answers in the spaces provided.

Vitreous humor

Pupil

Sclera

Lens

Retina

Cornea

1. _____

2. _____

3. _____

4. _____

5. _____

6. _____

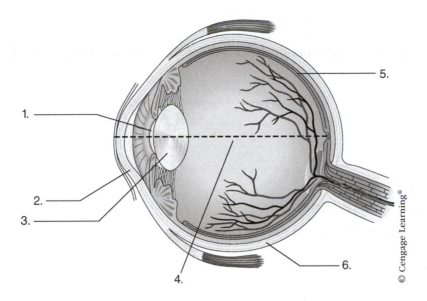

1.

2.

3.

4.

5.

6.

© Cengage Learning®

I. What Is This?

Read the statements that follow and identify the diagnostic technique, treatment, or procedure described. Write the appropriate answer in the space provided.

1. The lens of Mr. Nichols's eye has become progressively cloudy, losing its normal transparency, and has altered his perception of images due to the interference of light transmission to the retina. The ophthalmologist has scheduled Mr. Nichols for surgery to remove the anterior segment of the lens capsule along with the lens, allowing for the insertion of an intraocular lens implant. What is the name of this procedure? (hint: three words)

    _____

2. The ophthalmologist is performing a procedure on Ms. Blink to determine her risk for glaucoma. The patient's eyes are numbed for this test, which uses an ultrasonic-wave instrument to gauge the thickness of each cornea. What is the name of this test?

    _____

3. Susan Mead is having a procedure performed today to correct or reduce her nearsightedness (myopia). This is a surgical procedure in which a few layers of corneal surface cells are shaved off by an "excimer laser beam" to flatten the cornea and reduce myopia. What is the name of this procedure? (hint: three words)

    _____

4. Mr. Pate is attending a health fair at a local mall. An ophthalmology practice is performing a screening test for high intraocular pressure. The machine records deflections of the cornea from a puff of pressurized air and is the easiest method of testing children. What is the name of this test?

    Air-puff
    _____

5. Cindy Green is having reconstructive plastic surgery for the removal of a portion of the ear cartilage from each ear to bring the pinna and auricle nearer to her head. She is excited about having a normal appearance to her ears upon recovery. What is the name of this procedure?

    _____

J. Spelling

Identify the correct spelling of each medical term. Write the correct spelling in the space provided.

1. corneal   corneul   _____
2. hemianospia   hemianopsia   _____
3. keratoconis   keratoconus   _____
4. ophthalmologist   opthalmologist   _____
5. palpabral   palpebral   _____

K. Pronunciation to Spelling

Using the phonetic pronunciations that follow, spell the word correctly. Write your response in the space provided.

1. (**am**-blee-**OH**-pee-ah) _____
2. (**AY**-kwee-us) _____
3. (**ir**-id-oh-sigh-**KLEYE**-tis) _____
4. (oh-toh-**DIN**-ee-ah) _____
5. (tin-**EYE**-tus) _____

L. Construct-a-Word

Using the word elements that follow, construct words that match the definitions below. Be sure to drop the combining vowel when necessary. Write your response in the space provided.

labyrinth/o	-ptosis
blephar/o	-itis
ot/o	-opia
dacry/o	-itis
aden/o	-rrhea
dipl/o	

1. drooping of the upper eyelid _____
2. inflammation of the lacrimal (tear) gland _____
3. double vision _____
4. inflammation of the inner ear _____
5. drainage from the ear _____

CHAPTER 15

The Urinary System

A. Review Checkpoint: Anatomy & Physiology

Completion: Read each statement carefully and write the appropriate answer in the space provided.

1. The outer layer of the kidney (the cortex) contains millions of microscopic units called _____, which are the functional units of the kidneys.

2. The central collecting area of the kidney is known as the _____. (hint: two words)

3. The _____ are muscular tubes lined with mucous membrane, one leading from each kidney down to the urinary bladder.

4. The urinary _____ is a hollow muscular sac in the pelvic cavity that serves as a temporary reservoir for the urine.

5. The external opening of the urethra is called the _____. (hint: two words)

B. Review Checkpoint: Vocabulary

Build-a-Word: Test your word building skills. Using the clues below, build the appropriate medical terms.

1. Build a word that means "a substance that tends to inhibit the growth and reproduction of microorganisms"; pertaining to "against infection."

   _____ + _____ + _____ = _____
      against   infection   pertaining to   word

2. Build a word that means "an instrument that measures bladder capacity in relation to changing pressure"; "instrument used to measure the bladder."

   _____ + _____ + _____ = _____
      bladder or sac   vowel   instrument used to measure   word

3. Build a word that means "a kidney stone," also called a renal calculi.

   _____ + _____ + _____ = _____
      kidney   vowel   stone   word

4. Build a word that means "inflammation of the renal pelvis."

   _____ + _____ = _____
      renal pelvis   inflammation   word

5. Build a word that means "herniation of the urinary bladder," also known as a vesicocele.

   _____ + _____ + _____ = _____
      urinary bladder   vowel   herniation   word

C. Review Checkpoint: Word Elements

Matching: Match the word elements listed on the left to the appropriate definitions on the right.

_____ 1. azot/o
_____ 2. ket/o
_____ 3. vesic/o
_____ 4. olig/o
_____ 5. noct/i

a. urinary bladder
b. nitrogen
c. few, little, scanty
d. night
e. ketone bodies

D. Review Checkpoint: Common Signs and Symptoms

Matching: Match the sign or symptom on the left to the appropriate definition on the right.

_____ 1. anuria
_____ 2. enuresis
_____ 3. glycosuria
_____ 4. urgency
_____ 5. pyuria

a. a feeling of the need to void urine immediately
b. the presence of pus in the urine
c. the cessation (stopping) of urine production
d. bedwetting
e. abnormal presence of sugar in the urine

E. Review Checkpoint: Pathological Conditions

Completion: Read each statement carefully and write the appropriate answer in the space provided.

1. Inflammation of the urinary bladder is known as _____.

2. An inflammation of the glomerulus of the kidneys is called _____.

3. A group of clinical symptoms occurring when damage to the glomerulus of the kidney is present and large quantities of protein are lost through the glomerular membrane into the urine, resulting in severe proteinuria, is known as nephrotic syndrome or _____.

4. A hereditary disorder of the kidneys in which grapelike fluid-filled sacs or cysts replace normal kidney tissue is known as _____. (hint: three words)

5. Stone formations in the kidney is known as renal _____.

F. Review Checkpoint: Diagnostic Techniques, Treatments, and Procedures

Completion: Read each statement carefully and write the appropriate answer in the space provided.

1. The mechanical filtering process used to cleanse the blood of waste products, draw off excess fluids, and regulate body chemistry when the kidneys fail to function properly, using the peritoneal membrane as the filter, is known as _____. (hint: two words)

2. The surgical implantation of a healthy human donor kidney into the body of a patient with irreversible renal failure is known as _____. (hint: two words)

3. A blood test performed to determine the amount of urea and nitrogen (waste products normally excreted by the kidney) present in the blood is known as a(n) _____ test. (hint: three words)

4. The process of viewing the interior of the bladder using a cystoscope is called a(n) _____.

5. Also known as an excretory urogram, a(n) _____ is a radiographic procedure that provides visualization of the entire urinary tract: kidneys, ureters, bladder, and urethra, after a contrast dye is injected intravenously. (hint: two words)

G. Review Checkpoint: Common Abbreviations

Matching: Match the abbreviations on the left with the correct definitions on the right.

_____	1. ADH	a. continuous ambulatory peritoneal dialysis
_____	2. ESRD	b. glomerular filtration rate
_____	3. KUB	c. kidneys, ureters, bladder
_____	4. GFR	d. end-stage renal disease
_____	5. CAPD	e. antidiuretic hormone

H. Review Checkpoint: Putting It All Together

The following questions offer a review of the material studied in the urinary system. Read each question carefully and select, or write, the most appropriate answer.

1. An abnormal backflow (reflux) of urine from the bladder to the ureter is known as _____. (hint: two words)

2. A malignant tumor of the kidney occurring predominately in childhood is known as a(n) _____ tumor.

3. A malignant tumor of the kidney occurring in adulthood is known as renal cell _____.

4. A vague feeling of bodily weakness or discomfort, often marking the onset of disease or infection, is known as _____.

5. The state or quality of being indifferent, apathetic (without emotion), or sluggish is known as _____.

6. Which of the following terms means "abnormal presence of blood in the urine"?

   a. bacteriuria
   b. dysuria
   c. hematuria
   d. albuminuria

7. Which of the following terms means "painful urination"?

   a. bacteriuria
   b. dysuria
   c. hematuria
   d. albuminuria

8. Which of the following terms means "the presence of abnormally large quantities of protein in the urine"?

   a. bacteriuria
   b. dysuria
   c. hematuria
   d. albuminuria

9. Which of the following terms means "the act of eliminating urine from the body"?

   a. bacteriuria
   b. micturition
   c. ketonuria
   d. urinary retention

10. Which of the following terms means "cloudy"?

   a. turbid
   b. soluted
   c. dialysate
   d. radiopaque

11. Inflammation of the peritoneum is known as _____.

12. The depression, or pit, of an organ where the vessels and nerves enter is known as the _____.

13. The length of time the dialysis solution stays in the peritoneal cavity during peritoneal dialysis is known as the _____. (hint: two words)

14. The cup-shaped end of a renal tubule containing a glomerulus, also called the glomerular capsule, is known as _____. (hint: two words)

15. The medical term that means "without symptoms" is _____.

16. The smallest branch of an artery is known as a(n)

    a. calculus   c. arteriole
    b. calyx   d. meatus

17. The solution that contains water and electrolytes that passes through the artificial kidney to remove excess fluids and wastes from the blood, also called "bath," is known as

    a. dialysate   c. turbid
    b. nephrolith   d. residual urine

18. Urine that remains in the bladder after urination is known as

    a. azotemia   c. residual urine
    b. pyuria   d. albuminuria

19. Micturition is also known as

    a. voiding   c. bacteriuria
    b. a vesicocele   d. residual urine

20. Which of the following terms means "the presence of pus in the urine"?

    a. bacteriuria   c. uremia
    b. azotemia   d. pyuria

I. Labeling

Labeling 1

Using the terms listed below, label the following illustration of the urinary system by writing your answers in the spaces provided.

Urethral meatus

Urethra

Ureters

Right kidney

Renal cortex

1. _____

2. _____

3. _____

4. _____

5. _____

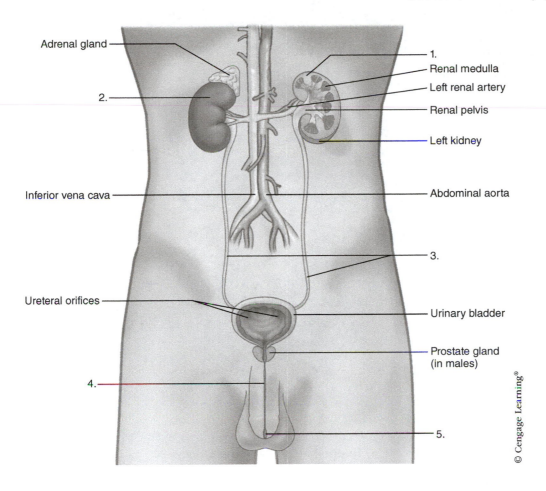

Adrenal gland

1.

Renal medulla

Left renal artery

Renal pelvis

2.

Left kidney

Inferior vena cava

Abdominal aorta

3.

Ureteral orifices

Urinary bladder

Prostate gland
(in males)

4.

5.

© Cengage Learning®

Labeling 2

Using the terms listed below, label the following illustration of the internal anatomy of the kidney by writing your answers in the spaces provided.

Renal pelvis

Medulla

Renal pyramid

Cortex

Ureter

Hilum

1. _____

2. _____

3. _____

4. _____

5. _____

6. _____

(continued)

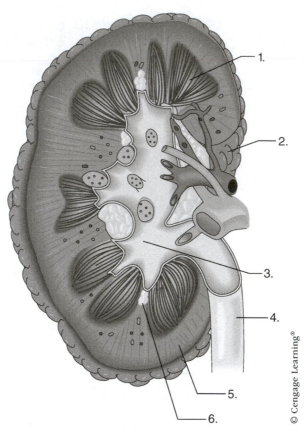

Internal anatomy of the kidney

J. What Is This?

Read the statements that follow and identify the diagnostic technique, treatment, or procedure described. Write the appropriate answer in the space provided.

1. Mr. Jones is suffering from end-stage renal disease. He has experienced a progressive irreversible deterioration in renal function, and his body is unable to maintain metabolic, fluid, and electrolyte balance. There is evidence of a progression toward uremia. Mr. Jones is frequently nauseated, is anorexic, has frequent episodes of hiccups, and has anemia. His physician has decided that it is time to provide a mechanical filtering process to cleanse the blood of waste products, draw off excess fluids, and regulate body chemistry for Mr. Jones. This will be accomplished using the peritoneal membrane as the filter. What is the name of this procedure? (hint: two words)

   _____

2. Mr. Jones is having difficulty with the CAPD treatment process because no one is at home (full-time) to assist him with the procedure. The doctor then decides to utilize another method to remove excess fluids and toxins from the blood by shunting Mr. Jones's blood from his body into a dialysis machine for filtering and then returning the clean blood to the patient's bloodstream. Mr. Jones will have to go to the dialysis unit three times a week for this procedure. What is the name of this procedure?

   _____

3. Mr. Jones has been receiving dialysis treatments for six months and was notified today that he is a match for a procedure that involves the surgical implantation of a healthy human donor kidney into his body (because of his irreversible renal failure). If this procedure is successful, kidney function will be restored and Mr. Jones will no longer be dependent on dialysis. What is the name of this procedure? (hint: two words)

   _____

4. George Flint is visiting the urologist today for complaints of urinary discomfort and generally not feeling well for quite some time. The doctor has ordered a test on Mr. Flint's urine and has requested a sterile specimen. The assistant will introduce a flexible hollow tube through Mr. Flint's urethra into the bladder to remove a sample of urine. What is the name of this procedure?

_____

5. Patti Payne is being seen by her urologist today for continued complaints of kidney stones. X-rays showed the presence of numerous small stones, which she passed, and the presence of a larger stone, which she has been unable to pass. The physician has decided to perform a noninvasive mechanical procedure using sound waves to break up the renal calculi so they can pass through the ureters. What is the name of this procedure? (hint: two words)

_____

K. Spelling

Identify the correct spelling of each medical term. Write the correct spelling in the space provided.

1. urethra   urether   _____

2. calix   calyx   _____

3. glomerulis   glomerulus   _____

4. polydispea   polydipsia   _____

5. bacteruria   bacteriuria   _____

L. Pronunciation to Spelling

Using the phonetic pronunciations that follow, spell the word correctly. Write your response in the space provided.

1. (**KAL**-kew-lus) _____

2. (**COR**-teks) _____

3. (dye-**AL**-ih-sis) _____

4. (**NEF**-roh-lith) _____

5. (**TER**-bid) _____

CHAPTER 16

The Male Reproductive System

A. Review Checkpoint: Anatomy & Physiology

Completion: Read each statement carefully and write the appropriate answer in the space provided.

1. The _____ is a tightly coiled tubule that resembles a comma and is the place where the sperm mature, becoming fertile and motile.

2. _____ is a combination of sperm and various secretions expelled from the body, through the urethra, during ejaculation (sexual intercourse).

3. The _____ gland lies just below the urinary bladder, where it surrounds the base of the urethra as it leaves the bladder.

4. The testicles are housed in the _____.

5. The specialized coils of tiny tubules within each testicle, which are responsible for production of sperm, are the _____. (hint: two words)

B. Review Checkpoint: Vocabulary

Build-a-Word: Test your word building skills. Using the clues below, build the appropriate medical terms.

1. Build a word that means "the surgical removal of the epididymis."

_____ + _____ = _____
   word root   suffix   word

2. Build a word that means "surgical fixation of an undescended testicle."

_____ + _____ + _____ = _____
   word root   combining vowel   suffix   word

3. Build a word that means "inflammation of the urethra."

_____ + _____ = _____
   word root   suffix   word

4. Build a word that means "an instrument used to view the rectum (has a cutting and cauterizing loop)."

_____ + _____ + _____ = _____
   word root   combining vowel   suffix   word

5. Build a word that means "the surgical removal of all or part of the prostate gland."

_____ + _____ = _____
   word root   suffix   word

C. Review Checkpoint: Word Elements

Matching: Match the word element listed on the left to the appropriate definition on the right.

_____ 1. cry/o

_____ 2. crypt/o

_____ 3. balan/o

_____ 4. orchid/o

_____ 5. andr/o

a. hidden

b. man, male

c. cold

d. glans penis

e. testicle

D. Review Checkpoint: Pathological Conditions

Completion: Read each statement carefully and write the appropriate answer in the space provided.

1. The absence of one or both testicles is known as _____.

2. A condition of undescended testicle(s); the absence of one or both testicles from the scrotum is known as _____.

3. An accumulation of fluid in any sac-like cavity or duct, particularly the scrotal sac or along the spermatic cord, is known as _____.

4. A congenital defect in which the urethra opens on the underside of the penis instead of at the end is known as _____.

5. A tightness of the foreskin (prepuce) of the penis that prevents it from being pulled back, creating some difficulty with urination, is known as _____.

E. Review Checkpoint: Diagnostic Techniques, Treatments, and Procedures

Completion: Read each statement carefully and write the appropriate answer in the space provided.

1. The process of viewing the interior of the bladder using a cystoscope is known as _____.

2. A(n) _____ is a surgical procedure in which the foreskin (prepuce) of the penis is removed.

3. An assessment of a sample of semen for volume, viscosity, sperm count, sperm motility, and percentage of any abnormal sperm is known as a(n) _____. (hint: two words)

4. The surgical removal of the prostate gland by making an incision into the abdominal wall, just above the pubic bone, is known as a(n) _____. (hint: two words)

5. The surgical removal of a portion of the prostate gland by inserting a resectoscope through the urethra and into the bladder is known as a(n) _____ of the prostate gland. (hint: two words)

F. Review Checkpoint: Common Abbreviations

Matching: Match the abbreviations on the left with the correct definitions on the right.

_____ 1. BPH

_____ 2. GU

_____ 3. KUB

_____ 4. PSA

_____ 5. IVP

a. intravenous pyelogram

b. kidneys, ureters, bladder

c. benign prostatic hypertrophy

d. genitourinary

e. prostate specific antigen

G. Review Checkpoint: Putting It All Together

The following questions offer a review of the material studied on the male reproductive system. Read each question carefully and select, or write, the most appropriate answer.

1. A skin lesion, usually of primary syphilis, that begins at the site of infection as a small raised area and develops into a red painless ulcer with a scooped-out appearance, also known as a venereal sore, is called a(n) _____.

2. The process of ejecting, or expelling, the semen from the male urethra is known as _____.

3. A loose, retractable fold of skin covering the tip of the penis, also called the prepuce, is known as the _____.

4. The area between the scrotum and the anus in the male and between the vulva and the anus in the female is known as the _____.

5. The singular form for the term that means "a mature male germ cell" is _____.

6. Which of the following terms means "weak; lacking normal muscle tone"?

   a. flaccid
   b. gonad
   c. dormant
   d. malaise

7. Which of the following terms means "the ability to move spontaneously"?

   a. flaccid
   b. motility
   c. vesicles
   d. dormant

8. Which of the following terms means "a vague feeling of bodily weakness or discomfort, often marking the onset of disease"?

   a. flaccid
   b. dormant
   c. prophylactic
   d. malaise

9. The narrow straight tube that transports sperm from the epididymis to the ejaculatory duct is the

   a. vas deferens
   b. bulbourethral gland
   c. prostate gland
   d. urethra

10. Inflammation of the glans penis and the mucous membrane beneath it is known as

    a. epididymitis
    b. urethritis
    c. balanitis
    d. phimosis

11. The inability of a male to achieve or sustain an erection of the penis is known as _____.

12. A congenital defect in which the urethra opens on the upper side of the penis at some point near the glans is known as _____.

13. Inflammation of the testes due to a virus, bacterial infection, or injury may affect one or both testicles. It typically results from the mump virus and is known as _____.

14. An abnormal dilation of the veins of the spermatic cord leading to the testicle is known as a(n) _____.

15. A benign enlargement of the prostate gland, creating pressure on the upper part of the urethra or neck of the bladder (causing obstruction of the flow of urine), is known as _____. (hint: three words)

16. Benign prostatic hypertrophy is a common condition occurring in men over the age of

    a. 50
    b. 40
    c. 35
    d. 25

17. The most common cause of cancer among men, and the most common cause of death due to cancer in men over the age of 55, is

    a. carcinoma urethra
    b. carcinoma of the prostate
    c. cancer of the epididymis
    d. cancer of testes

18. A protrusion of a part of the intestine through a weakened spot in the muscles and membranes of the inguinal region of the abdomen, in which the intestine pushes into and sometimes fills the entire scrotal sac in the male, is known as a(n)

    a. varicocele
    b. vesicocele
    c. inguinal hernia
    d. phimosis

19. A sexually transmitted bacterial infection that causes inflammation of the cervix (cervicitis) in women and inflammation of the urethra (urethritis) and epididymis (epididymitis) in men is known as

    a. chlamydia
    b. genital herpes
    c. gonorrhea
    d. genital warts

20. _____ is a highly contagious viral infection of the male and female genitalia, caused by the herpes simplex virus and transmitted by direct contact with infected body secretions; it can recur spontaneously once the virus has been acquired.

    a. chlamydia
    b. gonorrhea
    c. genital herpes
    d. syphilis

H. Labeling

Using the terms listed below, label the following illustration of the male reproductive system by writing your answers in the spaces provided.

Testis

Scrotum

Glans penis

Urethra

Prostate gland

1. _____

2. _____

3. _____

4. _____

5. _____

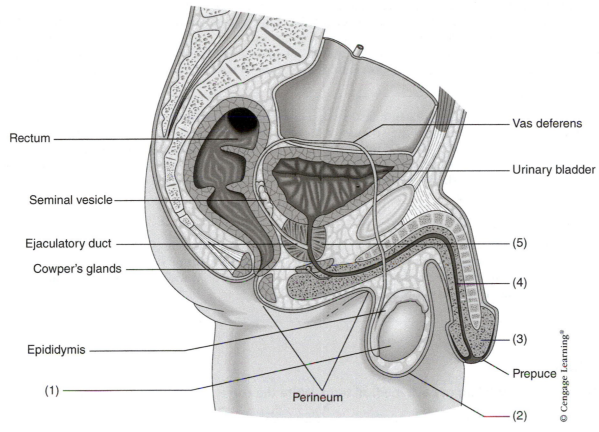

Rectum

Seminal vesicle

Ejaculatory duct

Cowper's glands

Epididymis

(1)

Perineum

Vas deferens

Urinary bladder

(5)

(4)

(3)

Prepuce

(2)

© Cengage Learning®

Male reproductive system

I. What Is This?

Read the statements that follow and identify the diagnostic technique, treatment, or procedure described. Write the appropriate answer in the space provided.

1. Dr. Knight is seeing a male patient today for complaints of dysuria, urinary frequency, and inflammation of the urethra. The patient is concerned that he may have contracted a sexually transmitted disease from an unidentified woman. Although most men are asymptomatic, the doctor suspects that the patient may have trichomoniasis. To confirm his suspicions, Dr. Knight will perform a microscopic examination of urethral secretions from his patient. A specimen of fresh urethral secretions will be placed on two separate clean microscopic slides and a drop of normal saline will be placed on top of one specimen, with a drop of potassium hydroxide placed on the other specimen. The slide will be placed under the microscope and observed for the presence of living organisms. What is the name of this procedure? (hint: two words)

_____

2. Dr. House has ordered a blood test for his male patient who is seeing him today due to the presence of a small, painless, red pustule on his penis (a chancre). The patient has confirmed sexual activity within the last two weeks. Dr. House suspects that his patient has syphilis and has ordered a microscopic examination of a smear taken from the lesion and a screening test for the presence of antibodies in his patient's blood. What is the acronym for this serological test for syphilis?

_____

3. Mr. and Mrs. Matthews have six children and do not wish to have any more. Since Mr. Matthews is 10 years older than Mrs. Matthews, he has decided to have a male sterilization in case anything should ever happen to him and she should ever remarry and want another child. The doctor has scheduled Mr. Matthews for a procedure that involves a surgical cutting and tying of the vas deferens to prevent the passage of sperm, consequently preventing pregnancy. What is the name of this procedure?

_____

4. Mr. Matthews had a male sterilization last week. His physician wants him to come back to the office for an additional test to confirm the success of the procedure. This test is an assessment of a sample of semen for volume, viscosity, sperm count, sperm motility, and percentage of any abnormal sperm. If the test does not confirm the absence of sperm, it will be repeated until sterility is confirmed. When two separate semen samples show no evidence of sperm, the man is considered sterile. What is the name of this test? (hint: two words)

_____

5. Mr. Gonzales has been diagnosed with benign prostatic hypertrophy. His condition has not responded to medical treatment, and the doctor has scheduled Mr. Gonzales for surgery. The doctor plans to surgically remove the prostate gland by making an incision into the abdominal wall, just above the pubic bone. What is the name of this procedure? (hint: two words)

_____

J. Spelling

Identify the correct spelling of each medical term. Write the correct spelling in the space provided.

1. semin   semen   _____

2. chancre   chanker   _____

3. epididymus   epididymis   _____

4. malodorous   malodrous   _____

5. vas defrens   vas deferens   _____

K. Pronunciation to Spelling

Using the phonetic pronunciations that follow, spell the word correctly. Write your response in the space provided.

1. (**ay**-simp-toh-**MAT**-ik) _____

2. (**or**-kee-oh-**PECK**-see) _____

3. (pal-**PAY**-shun) _____

4. (**ep**-ih-**DID**-ih-mis) _____

5. (**FLAK**-sid) _____

L. Construct-a-Word

Using the word elements that follow, construct words that match the meanings below. Be sure to drop the combining vowel when necessary. Write your response in the space provided.

dys-	orchi/o	-uria
an-	prostat/o	-pexy
	urethr/o	-ectomy
	orch/o	-itis
		-ism

1. surgical fixation of an undescended testicle _____

2. surgical removal of all or part of the prostate gland _____

3. inflammation of the urethra _____

4. painful urination _____

5. absence of one or both testicles _____

CHAPTER 17

The Female Reproductive System

A. Review Checkpoint: Anatomy & Physiology

Completion: Read each statement carefully and write the appropriate answer in the space provided.

1. Collectively, the external genitalia are referred to as the vulva or _____.

2. The _____ is the fatty tissue that covers and cushions the symphysis pubis. (hint: two words)

3. The _____ is a pear-shaped, hollow, muscular organ that houses the fertilized implanted ovum as it develops throughout pregnancy.

4. The uterine tubes, or oviducts, serve as a passageway for the ova (eggs) as they exit the ovary en route to the uterus and are also known as the _____ (hint: two words)

5. Also known as the female gonads, the _____ are the female sex cells.

B. Review Checkpoint: Vocabulary

Build-a-Word: Test your word building skills. Using the clues below, build the appropriate medical terms.

1. Build a word that means "the inner lining of the uterus."

   _____ + _____ + _____ = _____
       prefix   word root   suffix   word

2. Build a word that means "one who specializes in the study of diseases and disorders of the female reproductive system."

   _____ + _____ + _____ = _____
     word root   combining vowel   suffix   word

3. Build a word that means "surgical removal of the breast, as a treatment method for breast cancer."

   _____ + _____ = _____
     word root   suffix   word

4. Build a word that means "the muscular layer of the uterine wall."

   _____ + _____ + _____ + _____ = _____
   word root   combining form   word root   suffix   word

5. Build a word that means "pertaining to the female breasts."

   _____ + _____ = _____
     word root   suffix   word

C. Review Checkpoint: Word Elements

Matching: Match the word elements listed on the left to the appropriate definition on the right.

____	1. ante-	a.	breast
____	2. colp/o	b.	before; in front
____	3. hyster/o	c.	fallopian tubes
____	4. mast/o	d.	uterus
____	5. salping/o	e.	vagina

D. Review Checkpoint: Common Signs and Symptoms

Matching: Match the sign or symptom on the left to the appropriate definition on the right.

____	1. amenorrhea	a.	abnormally long or very heavy menstrual periods
____	2. dysmenorrhea	b.	absence of menstrual flow
____	3. menorrhagia	c.	abnormally light or infrequent menstruation
____	4. metrorrhagia	d.	painful menstrual flow
____	5. oligomenorrhea	e.	uterine bleeding at times other than the menstrual period

E. Review Checkpoint: Pathological Conditions

Completion: Read each statement carefully and write the appropriate answer in the space provided.

1. An acute or chronic inflammation of the uterine cervix is known as _____.

2. Herniation or downward protrusion of the urinary bladder through the wall of the vagina is known as _____.

3. The presence and growth of endometrial tissue in areas outside the endometrium (lining of the uterus) is known as _____.

4. Inflammation of the fallopian tubes, also known as salpingitis, is called _____. (hint: three words)

5. The inflammation of the vagina and the vulva is known as _____.

F. Review Checkpoint: Diagnostic Techniques, Treatments, and Procedures

Completion: Read each statement carefully and write the appropriate answer in the space provided.

1. A procedure in which the woman examines her breasts and surrounding tissue on a monthly basis for evidence of any changes that could indicate the possibility of malignancy is known as breast _____. (hint: two words)

2. The visual examination of the vagina and cervix with a colposcope is known as a(n) _____.

3. The surgical removal of a cone-shaped segment of the cervix for diagnosis or treatment is known as a cone biopsy or _____.

4. The destruction of tissue by rapid freezing with substances such as liquid nitrogen is known as _____.

5. The process of examination with X-ray the soft tissue of the breast to detect various benign and/or malignant growths before they can be felt is known as _____.

G. Review Checkpoint: Common Abbreviations

Matching: Match the abbreviations on the left with the correct definitions on the right.

____ 1. ECC   a. endocervical curettage

____ 2. HSG   b. hysterosalpingography

____ 3. HPV   c. carcinoma in situ

____ 4. LMP   d. human papilloma virus

____ 5. CIS   e. last menstrual period

H. Review Checkpoint: Putting It All Together

The following questions offer a review of the material studied on the female reproductive system. Read each question carefully and select, or write, the most appropriate answer.

1. The vaginal erectile tissue (structure) corresponding to the male penis is the _____.

2. One of the female hormones that promotes the development of the female secondary sex characteristics is _____.

3. The dome-shaped central, upper portion of the uterus between the points of insertion of the fallopian tubes is known as the _____.

4. The onset of menstruation, or the first menstrual period, is known as _____.

5. Another name for menstruation or menstrual flow is _____.

6. Which of the following terms means the permanent cessation (stopping) of the menstrual cycles?

     a. menarche   c. menorrhagia
     b. menopause   d. coitus

7. Which of the following terms is another name for sexual intercourse?

     a. coitus   c. fourchette
     b. climacteric   d. fertilization

8. A thin layer of elastic, connective tissue membrane that forms a border around the outer opening of the vagina and may partially cover the vaginal opening is known as the

     a. labia majora   c. hymen
     b. labia minora   d. fourchette

9. The periodic shedding of the lining of the nonpregnant uterus through a bloody discharge that passes through the vagina to the outside of the body, occurring at monthly intervals and lasting for 3 to 5 days, is known as

     a. mastitis   c. climacteric
     b. menstruation   d. ovulation

10. Which of the following terms refers to the muscular layer of the uterine wall?

     a. endometrium   c. myometrium
     b. perineum   d. diaphragm

11. The fringe-like end of the fallopian tube is known as the _____.

12. The medical term for menstrual flow or menstruation is _____.

13. The release of the mature ovum from the ovary, occurring approximately 14 days prior to the beginning of menses, is called _____.

14. *PMS* is the abbreviation for _____.

15. The period of life in which the ability to reproduce begins—in females, it is the period when the female reproductive organs are fully developed—is known as _____.

16. Which of the following terms refers to an opening or tunnel through any part of the body?

    a. meatus
    b. hymen

    c. cul-de-sac
    d. adnexa

17. Which of the following terms refers to the entrance or outlet of any body cavity?

    a. hymen
    b. hilum

    c. orifice
    d. adnexa

18. Which of the following terms means abstaining from having vaginal intercourse?

    a. coitus
    b. copulation

    c. abstinence
    d. climacteric

19. A thin, flexible square patch that continuously delivers hormones through the skin and into the bloodstream for a full seven days to prevent pregnancy is known as the

    a. birth control patch
    b. Depo-Provera

    c. intrauterine device
    d. extrauterine device

20. Another name for the vaginal orifice (opening) is vaginal

    a. labia majora
    b. introitus

    c. labia minora
    d. hymen

I. Labeling

Labeling 1

Using the terms listed below, label the following illustration of the external genitalia of the female reproductive system by writing your answers in the spaces provided.

Mons pubis

Labia majora

Perineum

Urinary orifice

Clitoris

1. _____

2. _____

3. _____

4. _____

5. _____

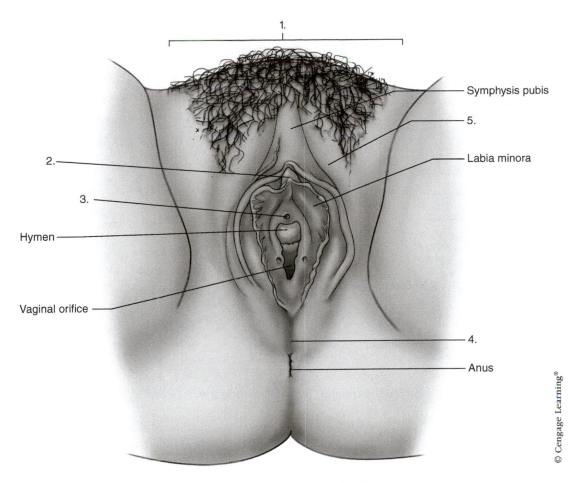

External genitalia, female reproductive system

Labeling 2

Using the terms listed below, label the following illustration of the internal genitalia of the female reproductive system by writing your answers in the spaces provided.

Fimbriae

Vagina

Ovary

Uterus

Fundus

Fallopian tube

1. _____

2. _____

3. _____

4. _____

5. _____

6. _____

(continued)

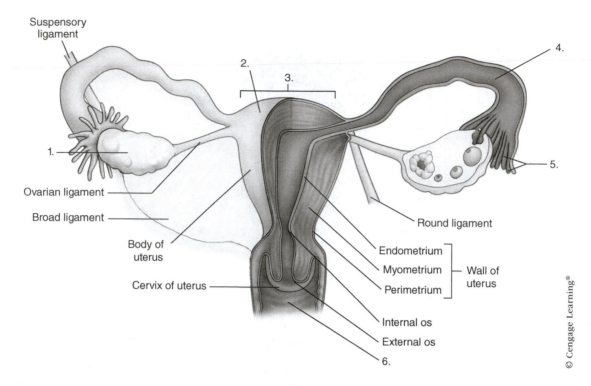

Internal genitalia, female reproductive system

J. What Is This?

Read the statements that follow and identify the diagnostic technique, treatment, or procedure described. Write the appropriate answer in the space provided.

1. Lisa Ingles is having her annual gynecological examination today. After the lab work and breast examination, the doctor has ordered a diagnostic test for cervical cancer. This is a microscopic examination of cells scraped from within the cervix, from around the cervix, and from the posterior part of the vagina. The secretions are smeared onto separate clean microscope slides and are "set" with a spray fixative. The slides are appropriately identified and will be sent to the lab for examination and interpretation by a pathologist. What is the name of this test? (hint: two words)

   _____

2. Candice Potts is having her annual gynecological examination today. Her physician is using a newer method of collecting a cervical cytology sample. The physician is using a process of collecting a tissue sample from the endocervix and the exocervix with a sampling device that is placed directly into a liquid fixative instead of being spread onto a glass slide. This process provides immediate fixation and improves specimen adequacy. What is the name of this procedure? (hint: three words)

   _____

3. Suzie Chung has discovered a lump in her breast. She is very upset and scared. Her physician has scheduled Suzie for an X-ray examination of the soft tissue of the breast. During this examination, the breast tissue is compressed between two clear disks for each X-ray view. The first view requires compressing the breast from top to bottom to take a top-to-bottom view (craniocaudal). The second view requires compressing the breast from side to side to take a mediolateral view. What is the name of this procedure?

   _____

4. Maggie Smith's recent Pap smear results indicate mild cervical dysplasia. Her physician has scheduled her for an in-office procedure that is used to remove abnormal cells from the surface of the cervix using a thin wire loop that acts like a scalpel. A painless electrical current passes through the loop as it cuts away a thin layer of surface cells from the cervix. The tissue specimen will be sent to a lab for evaluation and confirmation of a diagnosis. What is the abbreviation for this procedure?

_____

5. Maria Mendez is experiencing abnormal uterine bleeding. Her physician has scheduled Maria for a procedure in which a surgical puncture is made through the posterior wall of the vagina into the cul-de-sac to withdraw intraperitoneal fluid for examination. During the procedure, a culdoscope will be inserted into the cul-de-sac to visualize the area for any evidence of inflammation, purulent drainage, bleeding, ovarian cysts, ectopic pregnancy, or ovarian malignancy. Once the needle has been inserted into the area, fluid will be aspirated for examination. What is the name of this procedure?

_____

K. Spelling

Identify the correct spelling of each medical term. Write the correct spelling in the space provided.

1. mastectomy   masectomy   _____

2. fallopian tubes   faloppian tubes   _____

3. menstruation   menustration   _____

4. menorrhea   menarrhea   _____

5. adenexa   adnexa   _____

L. Pronunciation to Spelling

Using the phonetic pronunciations that follow, spell the word correctly. Write your response in the space provided.

1. (add-**NEK**-sah) _____

2. (ah-**REE**-oh-lah) _____

3. (**FIM**-bree-ay) _____

4. (**gigh**-neh-**KOL**-oh-jee) _____

5. (meh-**NAR**-kee) _____

Obstetrics

A. Review Checkpoint: Physiological Changes During Pregnancy

Completion: Read each statement carefully and write the appropriate answer in the space provided.

1. The most obvious changes in the uterine cervix are those of color and consistency. After approximately the sixth week of pregnancy, the cervix and vagina take on a bluish-violet hue as a result of the local venous congestion. This is known as _____ sign.

2. The softening of the cervix in preparation for childbirth is known as _____ sign.

3. The thin, yellowish discharge from the nipples throughout the pregnancy, which is a forerunner of breast milk, is known as _____.

4. The hyperpigmentation that appears on the abdomen of the pregnant female is seen as a darkened vertical midline between the fundus and the symphysis pubis, and is known as the _____. (hint: two words)

5. During the second half of pregnancy, a woman may experience stretch marks on the abdomen, thighs, and breasts; this is known as _____. (hint: two words)

B. Review Checkpoint: Vocabulary

Build-a-Word: Test your word building skills. Using the clues below, build the appropriate medical terms.

1. Build a word that means "a surgical incision into the woman's perineum to enlarge the vaginal opening for delivery of the baby"; literally "incision into the vulva."

   _____ + _____ + _____ = _____
   word root   vowel   suffix   word

2. Build a word that means a "forward curvature of the spine, noticeable if the person is observed from the side"; literally "condition of being bent."

   _____ + _____ = _____
   word root   suffix   word

3. Build a word that means "a special stethoscope for hearing the fetal heartbeat through the mother's abdomen."

   _____ + _____ + _____ = _____
   word root   vowel   suffix   word

4. Build a word that means "the branch of medicine that specializes in the treatment and care of the diseases and disorders of the newborn through the first four weeks of life."

   _____ + _____ + _____ + _____ = _____
   prefix   word root   vowel   suffix   word

5. Build a word that means "a woman who is pregnant for the first time."

_____ + _____ = _____
      word root   suffix   word

C. Review Checkpoint: Word Elements

Matching: Match the word elements listed on the left to the appropriate definition on the right.

_____ 1. -cyesis

_____ 2. episi/o

_____ 3. -salping/o

_____ 4. obstetr/o

_____ 5. -tocia

a. midwife

b. labor

c. pregnancy

d. vulva

e. fallopian tubes

D. Review Checkpoint: Complications of Pregnancy

Matching: Match the complication of pregnancy listed on the left to the appropriate definition on the right.

_____ 1. abortion

_____ 2. abruptio placenta

_____ 3. ectopic pregnancy

_____ 4. hyperemesis gravidarum

_____ 5. placenta previa

a. the premature separation of a normally implanted placenta from the uterine wall after the pregnancy has passed 20 weeks' gestation or during labor

b. termination of a pregnancy before the fetus has reached a viable age

c. a condition in which the placenta is implanted in the lower part of the uterus and precedes the fetus during the birthing process

d. abnormal implantation of a fertilized ovum outside the uterine cavity

e. an abnormal condition of pregnancy characterized by severe vomiting that results in maternal dehydration and weight loss

E. Review Checkpoint: Signs and Symptoms of Labor

Completion: Read each statement carefully and write the appropriate answer in the space provided.

1. Mild, irregular contractions that occur throughout pregnancy, sometimes mistaken for true labor, are known as _____ contractions. (hint: two words)

2. Occurring a few weeks prior to the onset of labor and as a result of the softening, dilation, and thinning of the cervix, the pregnant female will experience a vaginal discharge that is a mixture of thick mucus and pink or dark brown blood. This is known as the _____. (hint: two words)

3. The expectant mother will notice that she can breathe easier because the descent of the baby relieves some of the pressure from her diaphragm. When _____ occurs, most expectant mothers will refer to it by saying that the baby has "dropped."

4. The rupture of the double-layered sac that contains the fetus and the amniotic fluid during pregnancy is known as the rupture of the _____ sac.

5. Some women experience a(n) _____ shortly before the onset of labor. These women may suddenly have the energy to do major housecleaning duties—things they had not had the energy to do previously. They should be cautioned against this so they will not be fatigued when labor actually begins. (hint: four words)

F. Review Checkpoint: Diagnostic Techniques, Treatments, and Procedures

Completion: Read each statement carefully and write the appropriate answer in the space provided.

1. A surgical puncture of the amniotic sac for the purpose of removing amniotic fluid is known as a(n) _____.

2. A stress test used to evaluate the ability of the fetus to tolerate the stress of labor and delivery is known as an oxytocin challenge test or a _____. (hint: three words)

3. The use of an electronic device to monitor the fetal heart rate and the maternal uterine contractions is known as _____. (hint: two words)

4. A noninvasive procedure that uses high-frequency sound waves to examine internal structures and contents of the uterus is known as a(n) _____. (hint: two words)

5. The process of measuring the female pelvis, manually or by X-ray, to determine its adequacy for childbearing is known as _____.

G. Review Checkpoint: Common Abbreviations

Matching: Match the abbreviations on the left with the correct definitions on the right.

_____ 1. AFP   a. labor and delivery

_____ 2. EDD   b. spontaneous vaginal delivery

_____ 3. LNMP   c. alpha-fetoprotein

_____ 4. SVD   d. last normal menstrual period

_____ 5. L&D   e. expected date of delivery

H. Review Checkpoint: Putting It All Together

The following questions offer a review of the material studied in the chapter on obstetrics. Read each question carefully and select, or write, the most appropriate answer.

1. A physician who has had extensive training in the field of high-risk obstetrics and is concerned with the care of the mother and fetus at higher-than-normal risk for complications is known as a(n) _____.

2. The temporary organ of pregnancy that provides for fetal respiration, nutrition, and excretion and that is attached to the wall of the uterus is known as the _____.

3. The _____ consists of intertwined arteries and veins that arise from the center of the placenta and attaches to the navel of the fetus. It serves as the lifeline between the mother and the fetus, becoming the means of transport for the nutrients and waste products to and from the developing baby. (hint: two words)

4. Following childbirth, the placenta is known as the _____.

5. Fertilization, or _____, occurs when a sperm comes in contact with and penetrates a mature ovum.

6. A presumptive sign of pregnancy, movement of the fetus felt by the mother, occurring about 18 to 20 weeks' gestation and described as a faint abdominal fluttering, is known as

     a. ballottment   c. lightening

     b. quickening   d. effacement

7. Softening of the lower segment of the uterus is known as

    a. Braxton Hicks contractions   c. Hegar's sign
    b. Goodell's sign   d. Nagele's sign

8. A technique of using the examiner's finger to tap against the uterus, through the vagina, to cause the fetus to "bounce" within the amniotic fluid and feeling it rebound quickly is known as

    a. Braxton Hicks contractions   c. effacement
    b. ballottment   d. Nagele's sign

9. A special stethoscope for hearing the fetal heartbeat through the mother's abdomen is a

    a. fetoscope   c. laparoscope
    b. periscope   d. pelvimeter

10. The date of birth can be determined by subtracting three months from the beginning of the last normal menstrual period and adding one year and seven days to the date. This is known as

    a. Goodell's rule   c. Nagele's rule
    b. Hegar's rule   d. Chadwick's rule

11. Patches of tan or brown pigmentation associated with pregnancy, occurring mostly on the forehead, cheeks, and nose, is called _____ or the "mask of pregnancy."

12. The inner of the two membrane layers that surround and contain the fetus and the amniotic fluid during pregnancy is known as the _____.

13. The bluish-violet hue of the cervix and vagina after approximately the sixth week of pregnancy is known as _____ sign.

14. The thinning of the cervix, which allows it to enlarge the diameter of its opening in preparation for childbirth, occurring during the normal process of labor, is known as _____.

15. The term of pregnancy, or _____, equals 280 days from the onset of the last menstrual period, in which there is intrauterine development of the fetus from conception through birth.

16. Which of the following terms refers to the name given to the product of conception from the second through the eighth week of pregnancy?

    a. fetus   c. gamete
    b. embryo   d. gonad

17. Which of the following terms refers to the name given to the developing baby from approximately the ninth week after conception until birth?

    a. fetus   c. gamete
    b. embryo   d. gonad

18. Which of the following terms refers to the production and secretion of milk from the female breasts as nourishment for the infant?

    a. lactation   c. quickening
    b. lightening   d. leucorrhea

19. Which of the following terms refers to a woman who has been pregnant more than once?

    a. primigravida   c. multigravida
    b. primipara   d. multipara

20. Which of the following terms refers to a woman who has never completed a pregnancy beyond 20 weeks' gestation?

    a. primipara   c. nullipara
    b. multipara   d. primigravida

I. Labeling

Using the terms listed below, label the following diagram of the uterine structures and the amniotic sac from the chapter on obstetrics by writing your answers in the spaces provided.

Cervix

Placenta

Chorion

Amnion

Uterus

1. _____

2. _____

3. _____

4. _____

5. _____

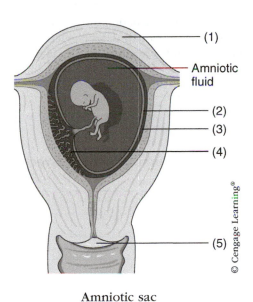

Amniotic sac

J. What Is This?

Read the statements that follow and identify the diagnostic technique, treatment, or procedure described. Write the appropriate answer in the space provided.

1. Mrs. Raymond is a 40-year-old primigravida. Because of her age and the fact that this is her first pregnancy, the doctor wants to perform a prenatal diagnostic test during the first trimester of Mrs. Raymond's pregnancy to check for possible Down syndrome in the unborn child. The procedure involves removing a small amount of placental tissue during the 11th to 13th week of pregnancy for genetic testing. What is the name of this procedure? (hint: three words)

_____

2. Mrs. Adams is four months' pregnant and is seeing her obstetrician for a routine visit today. During the visit, the physician notices that the fundal height measurement is in excess of normal. Knowing the Adams family history of multiple births, on both sides of the family, the doctor has ordered

a noninvasive procedure that uses high-frequency sound waves to examine the internal structures and contents of the uterus. This test can be used to detect very early pregnancy as well as the size and development of the fetus and is a valuable tool for diagnosis of multiple gestations. What is the name of this procedure? (hint: two words)

_____

3. Dr. Stark has scheduled her patient, Mrs. Cornwall, for a procedure today to determine the adequacy of her pelvis for childbearing. She has performed a clinical evaluation based on palpation of the bony landmarks in the pelvis and a mathematical estimate of the distance between them. Today she has ordered an X-ray of the pelvis to determine the dimensions of the bony pelvis of Mrs. Cornwall for a more definitive answer. What is the name of this procedure?

_____

4. The obstetrician has determined that her patient, Mrs. Juarez, does not have a pelvis of adequate size to deliver her baby vaginally. She estimates the baby's weight at nine pounds. The doctor has scheduled Mrs. Juarez for a surgical procedure in which the abdomen and uterus will be incised and the baby will be delivered transabdominally. This will be done shortly before her due date, as the doctor prefers that she not go into early labor. What is the name of this procedure? (hint: two words)

_____

5. Mrs. Rodriguez is 16 weeks' pregnant and is scheduled for a serum screening test for determining whether or not she might be at high risk for birth defects such as spina bifida, Down syndrome, or trisomy 18. This test is offered to pregnant women between 15 and 21 weeks' gestation. What is the abbreviation for this prenatal test?

_____ screening

K. Spelling

Identify the correct spelling of each medical term. Write the correct spelling in the space provided.

1. cesarean   caserean   _____

2. affacement   effacement   _____

3. fimbriae   fimbreia   _____

4. chloasma   choloasma   _____

5. umbilicle   umbilical   _____

L. Pronunciation to Spelling

Using the phonetic pronunciations that follow, spell the word correctly. Write your response in the space provided.

1. (sair-**KLAZH**) _____

2. (kloh-**AZ**-mah) _____

3. (con-**SEP**-shun) _____

4. (**FEET**-oh-skohp) _____

5. (nuh-**LIP**-ah-rah) _____

CHAPTER 19

Child Health

A. Review Checkpoint: Growth and Development

Completion: Read each statement carefully and write the appropriate answer in the space provided.

1. The physical increase in the whole or any of its parts is known as _____.

2. When measuring height or length, the infant is measured from the crown of the head to the _____.

3. _____ refers to the eruption of teeth and follows a sequential pattern.

4. _____ growth and development proceeds from head to toe.

5. Growth and development that proceeds from the center outward or from the midline to the periphery is known as _____ development.

B. Review Checkpoint: Vocabulary

Build-a-Word: Test your word building skills. Using the clues below, build the appropriate medical terms.

1. Build a word that means "pertaining to the armpit."

   _____ + _____ = _____
      word root   suffix   word

2. Build a word that literally means "one who specializes in new birth (a medical doctor)."

   _____ + _____ + _____ + _____ = _____
      prefix   word root   vowel   suffix   word

3. Build a word that means "inflammation of the navel."

   _____ + _____ = _____
      word root   suffix   word

4. Build a word that means "a physician who treats children."

   _____ + _____ = _____
      word root   suffix   word

5. Build a word that means "pertaining to the eardrum."

   _____ + _____ = _____
      word root   suffix   word

C. Review Checkpoint: Word Elements

Matching: Match the word elements listed on the left to the appropriate definition on the right.

_____ 1. cephal/o   a. child

_____ 2. epi-   b. head

_____ 3. nat/o   c. fire, heat

_____ 4. pedi/a   d. upon, over

_____ 5. pyr/o   e. birth

D. Review Checkpoint: Communicable Diseases

Matching: Match the word elements listed on the left to the appropriate definition on the right.

_____ 1. chickenpox

_____ 2. fifth disease

_____ 3. impetigo

_____ 4. mumps

_____ 5. pertussis

a. also known as whooping cough

b. characterized by successive eruptions of macules, papules, and vesicles on the skin; followed by crusting over of the lesions with a granular scab

c. also known as infectious parotitis

d. characterized by vesicles and pustules filled with millions of staphylococcus or streptococcus bacteria

e. characterized by a face that appears as "slapped cheeks"

E. Review Checkpoint: Pathological Conditions

Completion: Read each statement carefully and write the appropriate answer in the space provided.

1. _____ is a pervasive developmental disorder characterized by the individual being extremely withdrawn and absorbed with fantasy.

2. A congenital defect in which there is an open space between the nasal cavity and the lip, due to failure of the soft tissue and bones in this area to fuse properly during embryologic development, is known as _____. (hint: two words)

3. _____ is a childhood illness characterized by a barking cough, stridor, and laryngeal spasm.

4. _____ is a serious form of child abuse that describes a group of unique symptoms resulting from repetitive, violent shaking. (hint: three words)

5. The completely unexpected and unexplained death of an apparently well, or virtually well, infant is known as "crib death" or _____. (hint: four words)

F. Review Checkpoint: Diagnostic Techniques, Treatments, and Procedures

Completion: Read each statement carefully and write the appropriate answer in the space provided.

1. A urine specimen collected from a child is known as a(n) _____ urine collection.

2. A(n) _____ is a surgical procedure in which the foreskin of the penis is removed.

3. The foreskin of the penis is also known as the _____.

4. A(n) _____ is a method of obtaining a blood sample from a newborn or premature infant by making a shallow puncture of the lateral or medial area of the plantar surface of the heel. (hint: two words)

5. When collecting a urine specimen using a disposable urine collection bag, the bag is applied to the _____ area of the infant so that urine can collect in the bag for a specimen.

G. Review Checkpoint: Common Abbreviations

Matching: Match the abbreviations on the left with the correct definition on the right.

_____ 1. DS   a. tuberculosis

_____ 2. RDS   b. shaken baby syndrome

_____ 3. SBS   c. tetanus and diphtheria toxoid

_____ 4. Tb   d. Down syndrome

_____ 5. Td   e. respiratory distress syndrome

H. Review Checkpoint: Putting It All Together

The following questions offer a review of the material studied in the chapter on child health. Read each question carefully and select, or write, the most appropriate answer.

1. The field of medicine concerned with the development and care of children, specializing in the treatment and prevention of the diseases and disorders peculiar to children, is known as

   a. obstetrics   c. orthopedics
   b. pediatrics   d. neonatology

2. A registered nurse practitioner with advanced study and clinical practice in pediatric nursing is known as a PNP or

   a. pediatric nurse practitioner   c. parent nurse practitioner
   b. psychiatric nurse practitioner   d. physician's nurse practitioner

3. An important measurement because it is related to intracranial volume is known as

   a. length   c. head circumference
   b. weight   d. abdominal circumference

4. When measuring the length or height, the infant is measured from the crown of the head to the heel with the child in what position?

   a. prone   c. standing
   b. sitting   d. recumbent

5. This parent-completed method of at-home screening of infants and young children for developmental delays during the first five years of life has 30 items divided into five categories that are designed to assess the children in their natural environments. This developmental screening is the

   a. Ages & Stages Questionnaires (ASQ)   c. Denver Developmental Screening (DDS)
   b. Brazelton Neonatal Behavior Assessment (BNBA)   d. Dubowitz for Newborns

6. The baby teeth, first set of teeth, or primary teeth are also known as the _____ teeth.

7. A congenital anomaly characterized by abnormal smallness of the head in relation to the rest of the body and by underdevelopment of the brain, resulting in some degree of mental retardation, is known as _____.

8. A usually innate and permanent form of immunity to a specific disease is known as _____ immunity.

9. Inflammation of the umbilical stump, marked by redness, swelling, and purulent exudates in severe cases is known as _____.

10. The mean body temperature of a normal person as recorded by a clinical thermometer placed in the mouth is known as a(n) _____ temperature.

11. The newborn age span is defined as

   a. birth to 1 month
   b. 1 month to 1 year

   c. 1 year to 3 years
   d. 3 years to 6 years

12. The infancy age span is defined as

   a. birth to 1 month
   b. 1 month to 1 year

   c. 1 year to 3 years
   d. 3 years to 6 years

13. When a child uses the whole hand before picking up a small object between the thumb and forefinger, this is known as what pattern of development?

   a. cephalocaudal
   b. proximodistal

   c. general to specific
   d. simple to complex

14. What type of pulse is taken and the heart rate is heard with a stethoscope placed on the chest wall adjacent to the cardiac apex (top of the heart)?

   a. radial pulse
   b. apical pulse

   c. peripheral pulse
   d. pedal pulse

15. A common abnormal respiratory sound heard on auscultation of the chest during inspiration, characterized by discontinuous bubbling noises, is known as:

   a. crackles
   b. rales

   c. wheezing
   d. regurgitation

16. Another name for fever is _____.

17. An acute viral disease characterized by fever, swelling, and tenderness of one or more salivary glands—usually the parotid glands—is known as infectious parotitis, or _____.

18. Paroxysmal dyspnea (severe attack of difficult breathing), accompanied by wheezing caused by a spasm of the bronchial tubes or by swelling of the mucous membrane, is known as _____.

19. A condition of undescended testicle(s), or the absence of one or both testicles from the scrotum, is known as _____.

20. The medical term *talipes equinovarus* is also known as _____.

I. Labeling

Using the terms listed below, label the following diagram of the deciduous and permanent teeth by writing your answers in the spaces provided.

Central incisors (6–8 mo.)

Cuspid/canine (16–20 mo.)

Second molar (20–30 mo.)

First molar (10–16 mo.)

Lateral incisor (8–12 mo.)

1. _____

2. _____

3. _____

4. _____

5. _____

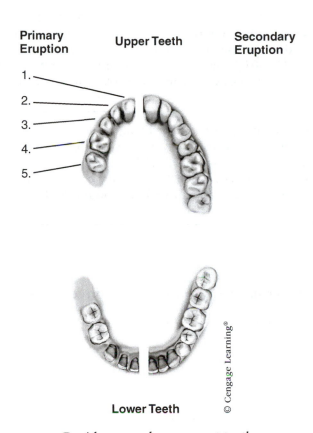

Primary Eruption	Upper Teeth	Secondary Eruption

1.
2.
3.
4.
5.

Lower Teeth

© Cengage Learning®

Deciduous and permanent teeth

J. What Is This?

Read the statements that follow and identify the communicable disease described. Write the appropriate answer in the space provided.

1. Mrs. Hughes brought her two-year-old son in to see the pediatrician today. The child woke up yesterday with a slight fever and eruptions of reddish blister-like areas on his abdomen and other areas of the body. Some of the areas have begun to crust over the lesions with a grainy type scab. Mrs. Hughes states that her son is constantly scratching the areas and she thinks she knows what he has, but she is not sure. What communicable disease do you think Mrs. Hughes's son has?

   _____

2. Susan Gonzales's daughter, Tina, attends a local day care center. Today, Ms. Gonzales brought Tina in to see the pediatrician because she has a superficial skin infection that has some blister-like areas that are draining—some are filled with pus. The lesions began on the face and spread after the child scratched the areas, and now she has many lesions. A couple of the lesions have scabbed over and have a honey-colored crust. What communicable disease do you think Ms. Gonzales's daughter has?

   _____

3. Mr. Parker has brought his son in to see the pediatrician today because the child woke up today with a fever and a rash all over the trunk of his body. His son doesn't seem to feel that bad, but Mr. Parker is concerned about the rash. The doctor has checked the child's throat and has determined that there are no spots in the area with grayish centers and red, irregular outer rings and the child's eyes are not sensitive to light. The doctor indicates what the child has and states that the rash should disappear in about three days and that the child should not return to school until about five days after the rash appeared. What communicable disease do you think Mr. Parker's son has?

_____

4. Ms. Nichols's daughter recently had a streptococcal infection and appeared to have recovered completely. Today, the child woke up with a sore throat, abrupt fever, a red and swollen tongue, and a point-like bright red rash on her body. This frightened Ms. Nichols and she has brought the child in to see the pediatrician. Based on these symptoms, what communicable disease do you think this child has?

_____

5. Mrs. Stanley's six-month-old daughter has run a fairly high fever for the last three days. Mrs. Stanley has been treating the fever with medication. Yesterday, the fever dropped and the temperature returned to normal, but the child had a rash all over the trunk of her body. Mrs. Stanley called the doctor to make an appointment and could be seen today. When Mrs. Stanley came to the pediatrician's office, the rash had almost disappeared. What communicable disease do you think Mrs. Stanley's daughter has?

_____

K. Spelling

Identify the correct spelling of each medical term. Write the correct spelling in the space provided.

1. axillary   axilliary   _____

2. decidius   deciduous   _____

3. febrile   febrill   _____

4. nomagram   nomogram   _____

5. statchure   stature   _____

L. Pronunciation to Spelling

Using the phonetic pronunciations that follow, spell the word correctly. Write your response in the space provided.

1. (**pee**-dee-ah-**TRISH**-an) _____

2. (im-**YOO**-nih-tee) _____

3. (om-fal-**EYE**-tis) _____

4. (tim-**PAN**-ik) _____

5. (**high**-droh-**SEFF**-ah-lus) _____

CHAPTER 20

Radiology and Diagnostic Imaging

A. Review Checkpoint: Radiology and Diagnostic Imaging Procedures and Techniques

Completion: Read each statement carefully and write the appropriate answer in the space provided.

1. A specialized diagnostic procedure in which a catheter is introduced into a large vein or artery and then threaded through the circulatory system to the heart is known as an angiocardiography or a(n) _____. (hint: two words)

2. The process of taking X-rays of the inside of a joint after a contrast medium has been injected into the joint is known as a(n) _____.

3. The infusion of a radiopaque contrast medium, barium sulfate, into the rectum to visualize the lower intestinal tract while X-ray films are obtained of the lower GI tract is known as a(n) _____. (hint: two words)

4. The oral administration of a radiopaque contrast medium, barium sulfate, which flows into the esophagus as a person swallows, is known as a(n) _____. (hint: two words)

5. The visualization of the gallbladder through X-ray following the oral ingestion of pills containing a radiopaque iodinated dye is known as a(n) _____.

6. Digital subtraction angiography is the process of providing images of _____ only, appearing without any background due to the use of a computerized digital video subtraction process. (hint: two words)

7. The diagnostic procedure in which ultrasound waves pass through the heart via a transducer, bounce off tissues of varying densities, and are reflected backward (or echoed) to the transducer—creating an image on the graph—is known as _____.

8. A radiological technique used to examine the function of an organ or a body part using a fluoroscope, and providing immediate serial images of the organ as it functions, is known as _____.

9. A noninvasive scanning procedure that provides visualization of fluid, soft tissue, and body structures using electromagnetic energy is known as _____. (hint: three words)

10. The process of taking X-rays of the soft tissue of the breast to detect various benign and/or malignant growths before they can be felt is known as _____.

B. Review Checkpoint: Vocabulary

Build-a-Word: Test your word building skills. Using the clues below, build the appropriate medical terms.

1. Build a word that means "the process of recording (or visualizing) the aorta."

   _____ + _____ + _____ = _____
     word root   vowel   suffix   word

2. Build a word that means "the process of recording the lymph vessels."

   _____ + _____ + _____ + _____ = _____
     word root   word root   vowel   suffix   word

3. Build a word that means "the process of recording the renal pelvis."

   _____ + _____ + _____ = _____
     word root   vowel   suffix   word

4. Build a word that means "one who records X-rays."

   _____ + _____ + _____ + _____ = _____
     word root   vowel   word root   suffix   word

5. Build a word that means "the study of radiation."

   _____ + _____ + _____ = _____
     word root   vowel   suffix   word

C. Review Checkpoint: Word Elements

Matching: Match the word elements listed on the left to the appropriate definition on the right.

____ 1. angi/o	a. pertaining to movement
____ 2. anter/o	b. bone marrow, spinal cord
____ 3. arthr/o	c. beyond
____ 4. cardi/o	d. front
____ 5. chol/e	e. joint
____ 6. cine-	f. bile
____ 7. fluor/o	g. vessel
____ 8. myel/o	h. heart
____ 9. ren/o	i. luminous
____ 10. ultra-	j. kidney

D. Review Checkpoint: Common Abbreviations

Completion: Read the abbreviations below and write the complete abbreviation in the space provided.

1. AP _____

2. Ba _____

3. DSA _____

4. ECHO _____

5. Fx _____

6. IVP _____

7. KUB _____

8. SBS _____

9. MRI _____

10. u/s _____

E. Review Checkpoint: Putting It All Together

The following questions offer a review of the material studied in the chapter on radiology and diagnostic imaging. Read each question carefully and select, or write, the most appropriate answer.

1. Movement of a limb away from the body is known as

   a. adduction
   b. abduction

   c. flexion
   d. extension

2. Movement of a limb toward the axis of the body is known as

   a. adduction
   b. abduction

   c. flexion
   d. extension

3. An X-ray view that has the beam directed from the front to the back of the body is known as

   a. posteroanterior
   b. lateral

   c. anteroposterior
   d. oblique

4. The filming with a movie camera of the images that appear on a fluorescent screen, especially those images of body structures that have been injected with a nontoxic radiopaque medium for diagnostic purposes, is known as

   a. cineradiography
   b. angiography

   c. computed tomography
   d. brachytherapy

5. A turning outward or inside out, such as a turning of the foot outward at the ankle, is known as

   a. flexion
   b. extension

   c. eversion
   d. plantar flexion

6. A movement allowed by certain joints of the skeleton that increases the angle between two adjoining bones is known as

   a. flexion
   b. extension

   c. eversion
   d. plantar flexion

7. A movement allowed by certain joints of the skeleton that decreases the angle between two adjoining bones is known as

   a. flexion
   b. extension

   c. eversion
   d. circumduction

8. A substance capable of causing death is said to be

   a. lethal
   b. palliative

   c. curative
   d. axial

9. A substance that soothes or relieves discomfort is said to be

   a. lethal
   b. palliative

   c. curative
   d. axial

10. When a person is lying facedown in a horizontal position, this person is in which position?

    a. recumbent

    b. lateral

    c. prone

    d. lithotomy

11. The abbreviation for *radiation absorbed dose*; the basic unit of absorbed ionizing radiation, is _____.

12. The term that means "pertaining to materials that allow X-rays to penetrate with a minimum of absorption" is _____.

13. The term that means "not permitting the passage of X-rays or other radiant energy is" _____.

14. Another name for roentgenology is _____.

15. When a patient is lying horizontally on the back, the position is known as _____.

16. The handheld device that sends and receives a sound-wave signal is a(n) _____.

17. An ultrasound is also known as a(n) _____.

18. The goal of therapy with radiation is to reach maximum tumor control with _____ normal tissue damage.

19. The X-ray of the _____ and the _____ (hint: two words) by injecting a contrast material into these structures is known as a hysterosalpingography.

20. The X-ray visualization of the bladder and urethra during the voiding process, after the bladder has been filled with a contrast material, is known as a voiding _____.

F. What Is This?

Read the statements that follow and identify the radiological and diagnostic imaging procedure or technique described. Write the appropriate answer in the space provided.

1. Mr. Pate is having a procedure that involves inserting a radiopaque catheter into the femoral artery. Using fluoroscopy, the catheter will be guided up the aorta to the level of the renal arteries. A contrast dye will be injected and a series of X-rays will be taken to visualize the renal vessels. The purpose of this procedure is to detect narrowing of the renal vessels, vascular damage, renal vein thrombosis, cysts, and/or tumors. What is the name of this procedure? (hint: two words)

   _____

2. Mr. Jeter is scheduled for an exam that involves visualizing and outlining of the major bile ducts following the intravenous injection of a contrast medium. The bile duct structure will be observed for obstruction, strictures, anatomic variations, malignant tumors, and congenital cysts during this procedure. This procedure is known as an intravenous _____.

   _____

3. Mrs. Jones fell and broke the tibial plateau of her left leg. Her orthopedist has ordered a noninvasive scanning procedure that provides visualization of fluid, soft tissue, and bony structures using electromagnetic energy, to determine the extent of the injury and the possible need for surgery. Mrs. Jones will be placed inside a large electromagnetic, tube-like machine where specific radio frequency signals change the alignment of hydrogen atoms in the body. The absorbed radio frequency energy will be analyzed by a computer and an image will be projected onto the screen for diagnosis. What is the name of this procedure? (hint: three words)

   _____

4. Mr. Medina is scheduled for a radiographic procedure that provides visualization of the entire urinary tract. A contrast dye will be injected intravenously and multiple X-rays films will be taken as the medium is cleared from the blood by glomeruli filtration of the kidney. This procedure is useful in diagnosing renal tumors, cysts, stones, structural or functional abnormalities of the bladder, and ureteral obstruction. What is the name of this procedure? (hint: two words)

_____

5. Mrs. Hill has been complaining of pain in the calf of her left leg. She is experiencing tenderness to the touch and warmness in the area. Her doctor has scheduled her for a procedure in which sound waves are transmitted into the body structures as a small transducer is passed over the skin. The physician will be checking for the possibility of deep vein thrombosis. The area to be examined will be lubricated before applying the transducer. As the sound waves are reflected back into the transducer, they will be interpreted by a computer, which presents the composite in a picture form. What is the name of this procedure?

_____

G. Spelling

Identify the correct spelling of each medical term. Write the correct spelling in the space provided.

1. brachytherapy brachitherapy _____

2. fluoroscopy floroscopy _____

3. myalography myelography _____

4. radiolusent radiolucent _____

5. anteroposterior anterioposterior _____

H. Pronunciation to Spelling

Using the phonetic pronunciations that follow, spell the word correctly. Write your response in the space provided

1. (ar-**THROG**-rah-fee) _____

2. (ee-**VER**-zhun) _____

3. (floo-**RES**-ens) _____

4. (**ray**-dee-**OL**-oh-jist) _____

5. (trans-**DOO**-sir) _____

I. Build-a-Word

Build a word that means:

1. radiation therapy administered by a machine positioned at some distance from the patient

   _____

2. pertaining to the kidney _____

3. X-ray of the bronchi after they have been coated with a radiopaque substance _____

4. process of X-raying the veins using a contrast medium _____

5. process of X-raying soft tissues of the breast _____

J. Match Point

Match the following abbreviations to the appropriate definition.

_____ 1. BE   a. computed tomography

_____ 2. CT   b. nothing by mouth

_____ 3. MRA   c. radioactive iodine

_____ 4. NPO   d. magnetic resonance angiography

_____ 5. RAI   e. barium enema

K. Construct a Word

Using the word elements that follow, construct words that match the meanings below. Be sure to drop the combining vowel when necessary. Write your response in the space provided.

radi/o	-grapher
lymph/o	-scopy
radi/o	-graphy
angi/o	-logist
fluor/o	-graphy
	bronch/o

1. X-ray examination of lymph glands and lymphatic vessels after an injection of contrast medium

   _____

2. one who specializes in the study of radiation (X-rays) _____

3. the process of viewing the function of an organ using a fluoroscope _____

4. X-ray examination of the bronchi after they have been coated with a radiopaque substance

   _____

5. one who takes, or records, X-rays _____

L. Is This the Same?

Read each question carefully and provide the most appropriate response. Record your response in the space provided.

1. Does *aortography* mean the same as *arthrography*?

   _____ Yes   _____ No

   If "No," which word means "a radiographic process of visualizing the inside of a joint using air or a contrast medium"?

   _____

2. Does *anteroposterior* mean the same as *posteroanterior*?

   _____ Yes   _____ No

   If "No," which word means "from the front to the back of the body"?

   _____

3. Does *abduction* mean the same as *adduction*?

   _____ Yes   _____ No

   If "No," which word means "movement of a limb away from the body"?

   _____

4. Does *radiology* mean the same as *roentgenology*?

   _____ Yes   _____ No

   If "No," which word means "the study of diagnostic and therapeutic uses of X-ray"?

   _____

5. Does *inversion* mean the same as *eversion*?

   _____ Yes   _____ No

   If "No," which word means "a turning outward"?

   _____

CHAPTER 21

Oncology (Cancer Medicine)

A. Review Checkpoint: Vocabulary

Completion: Read each statement carefully and write the appropriate answer in the space provided.

1. The medical specialty concerned with the study of malignancy is known as _____.

2. A change in the structure and orientation of cells characterized by a loss of specialization and reversion to a more primitive form is known as _____.

3. When a growth is enclosed in fibrous or membranous sheaths, it is said to be _____.

4. In radiology, the division of the total dose of radiation into small doses administered at intervals in an effort to minimize tissue damage is known as _____.

5. When a growth is characterized by a tendency to spread, infiltrate, and intrude, it is said to be _____.

6. Build a word that means "a cancerous tumor."

   _____ + _____ = _____
     word root   suffix   word

7. Build a word that means "excessive formation or growth."

   _____ + _____ = _____
       prefix   suffix   word

8. Build a word that means "abnormal formation or growth of any new tissue, benign or malignant."

   _____ + _____ = _____
       prefix   suffix   word

9. Build a word that means "tumor of the flesh (a malignant neoplasm of the connective and supportive tissues of the body)."

   _____ + _____ = _____
     word root   suffix   word

10. Build a word that means "that which generates cancer."

    _____ + _____ + _____ = _____
      word root   vowel   suffix   word

B. Review Checkpoint: Word Elements

Matching: Match the word elements listed on the left to the appropriate definition on the right.

_____ 1. -blast   a. tumor

_____ 2. cry/o   b. formation or growth

_____ 3. carcin/o   c. beyond, after

_____ 4. meta-   d. of or related to the flesh

_____ 5. -oma   e. cancer

_____ 6. -plasia   f. hard

_____ 7. sarc/o   g. cold

_____ 8. scirrh/o   h. upon

_____ 9. ana-   i. embryonic stage of development

_____ 10. epi-   j. not, without

C. Review Checkpoint: Classification of Neoplasms

Matching: Match the term listed on the left to the appropriate definition on the right.

_____ 1. benign tumor

_____ 2. malignant tumor

_____ 3. carcinoma

_____ 4. sarcoma

_____ 5. leukemias

a. occur in blood-forming organs such as the spleen and in the bone marrow

b. solid tumor that originates from epithelial tissue and internal body surfaces, the lining of blood vessels, body cavities, glands, and organs

c. is usually encapsulated

d. able to metastasize to distant sites through the blood or lymph systems

e. originates from supportive and connective tissue such as bone, fat, muscle, and cartilage

D. Review Checkpoint: Specific Types of Cancer

Completion: Read each statement carefully and write the appropriate answer in the space provided.

1. A malignant epithelial cell tumor that begins as a slightly elevated nodule with a depression or ulceration in the center that becomes more obvious as the tumor grows is known as a(n) _____ carcinoma. (hint: two words)

2. Bronchogenic carcinoma is a malignant lung tumor that originates in the bronchi; it is also known as _____ cancer.

3. In the earliest stage of cervical cancer, the cancer remains in place without spreading; it just sits there. This early stage of cervical cancer is known as carcinoma _____. (hint: two words)

4. A malignant tumor of the inner lining of the uterus, adenocarcinoma of the uterus, is also known as _____ carcinoma.

5. Rare malignant lesions that begin as soft purple-brown nodules or plaques on the feet and gradually spread through the skin, and has an increased incidence in individuals infected with AIDS, is known as _____ sarcoma.

6. A malignant skin tumor originating from melanocytes in preexisting moles, freckles, or skin with pigment—a darkly pigmented cancerous tumor—is known as a malignant _____.

7. A malignant tumor of the kidney, occurring in adulthood, is known as _____ carcinoma. (hint: two words)

8. A malignant tumor of the kidney occurring predominantly in childhood is known as a(n) _____ tumor.

9. The most frequently diagnosed cancer in men is _____ cancer.

10. A precancerous lesion occurring anywhere in the mouth, evidenced by elevated gray-white or yellow-white leathery surfaced lesions with clearly defined borders, is known as _____. (hint: two words)

E. Review Checkpoint: Diagnostic Treatment, Techniques, and Procedures

Completion: Read each statement carefully and write the appropriate answer in the space provided.

1. The use of cytotoxic drugs and chemicals to achieve a cure, decrease tumor size, provide relief of pain, or slow metastasis is known as _____.

2. An advanced treatment procedure for skin cancer in which the cancerous tumor is removed in stages, the tissue is examined for evidence of cancer, and additional tissue is removed until negative boundaries are confirmed is known as _____. (hint: two words)

3. The use of ionizing radiation to interrupt cellular growth by reaching maximum tumor control with minimum normal tissue damage is known as _____ therapy.

4. A biopsy that involves removing a piece of a tumor for examination and diagnosing is known as a(n) _____ biopsy.

5. The surgical procedure that involves a wide resection that removes the organ of origin and surrounding tissue is known as a(n) _____.

F. Review Checkpoint: Common Abbreviations

Matching: Match the abbreviations on the left with the correct definition on the right.

____ 1. Bx   a. biopsy

____ 2. Ca   b. cancer

____ 3. PSA   c. ribonucleic acid

____ 4. RNA   d. prostate-specific antigen

____ 5. mets   e. metastasis

G. Review Checkpoint: Putting It All Together

The following questions offer a review of the material studied in the chapter on oncology (cancer medicine). Read each question carefully and select or write the most appropriate answer.

1. Which of the following terms refers to an abnormal growth of new tissue that serves no useful purpose?

   a. differentiation
   b. neoplasm

   c. hypoplasia
   d. anaplasia

2. Which of the following terms means "a change in the structure and orientation of cells characterized by a loss of specialization and reversion to a more primitive form"?

   a. antimetabolite
   b. differentiation

   c. anaplasia
   d. benign

3. Which of the following terms refers to a substance or agent that causes the development or increases the incidence of cancer?

   a. carcinogen
   b. cytotoxic

   c. chemotherapy
   d. fractionation

4. Which of the following terms means "characterized by a tendency to spread, infiltrate, and intrude"?

   a. dedifferentiation
   b. fractionation

   c. invasive
   d. encapsulated

5. Which of the following terms means "surgical removal of only the tumor and the immediate adjacent breast tissue (a method of treatment for breast cancer when detected in the early stage of the disease)"?

   a. lumpectomy
   b. cryosurgery

   c. radical mastectomy
   d. exenteration

6. A type of cell division that results in the formation of two genetically identical daughter cells is known as _____.

7. The physician who specializes in the study and treatment of neoplastic diseases, particularly cancer, is called a(n) _____.

8. A written plan or description of the steps to be taken in a particular situation, such as conducting research, is known as the _____.

9. A patient who exhibits again the symptoms of a disease from which he/she appeared to have recovered is said to have a(n) _____.

10. The risk that refers to the probability that an individual, over the course of his or her lifetime, will develop cancer or will die from cancer, is known as the _____ risk.

11. A _____ carcinoma is the most common malignant tumor of the epithelial tissue, occurring most often on areas of the skin exposed to the sun (usually between the hairline and the upper lip).

   a. squamous cell
   b. basal cell

   c. renal cell
   d. neuroblastoma

12. The presence of a malignant neoplasm in the large intestine is known as

   a. colorectal cancer
   b. cervical cancer

   c. adenocarcinoma
   d. anal cancer

13. The U.S. Food and Drug Administration (FDA) has approved a vaccine that is highly effective in preventing infections from two high-risk HPVs that cause approximately _____% of cervical cancers and two HPVs that cause approximately _____% of genital warts.

   a. 70, 90
   b. 90, 60

   c. 80, 85
   d. 100, 90

14. The classic symptom of endometrial carcinoma is abnormal uterine _____.

    a. bleeding
    b. sluffing

    c. rippling
    d. stretching

15. A malignancy of the squamous cells of epithelial tissue, which is a much faster growing cancer than basal cell carcinoma and has a greater potential for metastasis if not treated, is known as _____ carcinoma.

    a. squamous cell
    b. basal cell

    c. renal cell
    d. neuroblastoma

16. Carcinoma of the testes is also known as _____ cancer.

17. The combining form *carcin/o* means _____.

18. The combining form *cry/o* means _____.

19. The prefix *meta-* means _____.

20. The suffix *-oma* means _____.

H. What Is This?

Read the statements that follow and identify the diagnostic technique, treatment, or procedure described. Write the appropriate answer in the space provided.

1. Ms. Ragan is scheduled for a procedure with her plastic surgeon. The surgeon will be performing a surgery that is an advanced treatment for skin cancer. During this procedure, the cancerous tumor will be removed in stages, the tissue will be examined for evidence of cancer, and additional tissue will be removed until negative boundaries are confirmed. This process will allow the surgeon to excise the tumor, remove layers of tissue, and examine the fresh tissue immediately, removing only tissue containing cancer and keeping the healthy tissue intact. What is the name of this procedure?

   _____

2. Ms. Tallent is scheduled to have a lesion removed from her arm. The physician will remove a piece of the tumor for examination and diagnosing. What is the name of this procedure? (hint: two words)

   _____

3. Ms. Winter is scheduled for a modified radical mastectomy. This procedure is also known by another name, in which the resection includes the removal of a tumor and a large area of surrounding tissue that contains lymph nodes. What is the other name for this procedure? (hint: two words)

   _____

4. Mr. White has been diagnosed with a malignant tumor. The physician plans treatment with the use of ionizing radiation to interrupt cellular growth, with the goal of reaching maximum tumor control with minimum normal tissue damage. What is the name of this treatment? (hint: two words)

   _____

5. Ms. Summers is being treated by her oncologist for cancer of the breast. The doctor plans to treat using surgery first, followed by the administration of cytotoxic drugs and chemicals, to achieve a cure, provide relief of pain, and slow the potential for metastasis. What is the name of this treatment method the doctor plans to use on Ms. Summers?

   _____

I. Spelling

Identify the correct spelling of each medical term. Write the correct spelling in the space provided.

1. metastasis   metastesis   _____

2. oncogenosis   oncogenesis   _____

3. cytotoxic   cytatoxic   _____

4. aduvant   adjuvant   _____

5. antineoplastic   antineaplastic   _____

J. Pronunciation to Spelling

Using the phonetic pronunciations that follow, spell the word correctly. Write your response in the space provided.

1. (**AD**-joo-vant) _____

2. (**an**-ah-**PLAY**-zee-ah) _____

3. (bee-**NINE**) _____

4. (kar-**SIN**-oh-jen) _____

5. (moh-**DAL**-ih-tee) _____

K. Construct-a-Word

Using the word elements that follow, construct words that match the meanings below. Be sure to drop the combining vowel when necessary. Write your response in the space provided.

hyper-	carcin/o	-oma
neo-	cyt/o	-ic
onc/o	-plasm	tox/o
-ia	plas/o	-genesis

1. a malignant tumor _____

2. pertaining to being destructive (poisonous) to cells _____

3. excessive formation or growth ("noun form") _____

4. any abnormal growth of new tissue, benign or malignant _____

5. the formation of a tumor _____

L. Is It the Same?

Read each question carefully and provide the most appropriate response. Record your response in the space provided.

1. Does *anaplasia* mean the same as *dedifferentiation*?

   _____ Yes   _____ No

   If "No," then which term means "a change in the structure and orientation of cells characterized by a loss of specialization and reversion to a more primitive form"?

   _____

2. Does *modality* mean the same as *morbidity*?

   _____ Yes   _____ No

   If "No," then which term means "a method of application (i.e., a treatment method)"?

   _____

3. Does *relapse* mean the same as *remission*?

   _____ Yes   _____ No

   If "No," then which term means "to exhibit again the symptoms of a disease from which a patient appears to have recovered"?

   _____

4. Does *verrucous* mean the same as *scirrhous*?

   _____ Yes   _____ No

   If "No," then which term means "rough, warty"?

   _____

5. Does *endometrial carcinoma* mean the same as *adenocarcinoma of the uterus*?

   _____ Yes   _____ No

   If "No," then which term means "malignant tumor of the inner lining of the uterus"?

   _____

CHAPTER 22

Pharmacology

A. Review Checkpoint: Vocabulary

Build-a-Word: Test your word building skills. Using the clues below, build the appropriate medical terms.

1. Build a word that means "pertaining to within a vein."

   _____ + _____ + _____ = _____
      prefix   word root   suffix   word

2. Build a word that means "pertaining to under the skin."

   _____ + _____ + _____ = _____
      prefix   word root   suffix   word

3. Build a word that means "the study of drugs, medicine."

   _____ + _____ + _____ = _____
     word root   vowel   suffix   word

4. Build a word that means "a specialist in drugs, medicine (one who is licensed to prepare and dispense drugs)."

   _____ + _____ = _____
     word root   suffix   word

5. Build a word that means "pertaining to under the tongue."

   _____ + _____ + _____ = _____
      prefix   word root   suffix   word

B. Review Checkpoint: Word Elements

Matching: Match the word elements on the left to the appropriate definition on the right.

_____ 1. esthesi/o   a. feeling, sensation

_____ 2. hypno-   b. sleep

_____ 3. lingu/o   c. tongue

_____ 4. or/o   d. mouth

_____ 5. ven/o   e. vein

C. Review Checkpoint: Routes of Administration for Medication

Completion: Read each statement carefully and write the appropriate answer in the space provided.

1. A(n) _____ medication is placed in the mouth next to the cheek.

2. A(n) _____ medication is one that is sprayed or inhaled into the nose, throat, and lungs.

3. A(n) _____ medication is one that is applied directly to the skin or mucous membrane for a local effect to the area.

4. A(n) _____ injection consists of injecting a small amount of medication just beneath the epidermis.

5. A(n) _____ injection consists of injecting the medication directly into large muscles.

D. Review Checkpoint: Drug Classifications

Matching: Match the drug classification on the left with the correct definition on the right.

_____ 1. analgesic   a. prevents or relieves nausea and vomiting

_____ 2. antibiotic   b. induces sleep or dulls the senses

_____ 3. antiemetic   c. relieves cough due to various causes

_____ 4. antitussive   d. relieves pain

_____ 5. hypnotic   e. stops or controls the growth of infection-causing microorganisms

E. Review Checkpoint: Common Charting Abbreviations

Completion: Read each statement carefully and write the appropriate answer in the space provided.

1. The abbreviation for "before meals" is _____

2. The abbreviation for "twice a day" is _____

3. The abbreviation for "milligram" is _____

4. The abbreviation for "over-the-counter drugs that require no prescription" is _____.

5. The abbreviation for "after meals" is _____

F. Review Checkpoint: Putting It All Together

The following questions offer a review of the material studied in the chapter on pharmacology. Read each question carefully and select or write the most appropriate answer.

1. The law requires that all preparations called by the same drug name must be of a uniform strength, quality, and purity. These rules that have been established to control the strength, quality, and purity of medications prepared by various manufacturers are known as

   a. references   c. controlled substances
   b. standards   d. package inserts

2. The body's reaction to a drug in an unexpected way that may endanger a patient's health and safety is known as what type of reaction?

   a. therapeutic   c. adverse
   b. desired   d. idiopathic

3. The name under which the drug is sold by a specific manufacturer, also known as the trade name, is the

   a. brand name
   b. generic name
   c. official name
   d. over-the-counter name

4. Any special symptom or circumstance that indicates the use of a particular drug or procedure is dangerous, is not advised, or has not been proven safe for administration is known as a

   a. cumulation
   b. therapeutic reaction
   c. contraindication
   d. local effect

5. The first dose of a medication is known as the

   a. initial dose
   b. therapeutic dose
   c. official dose
   d. standard

6. Medication injected directly into the vein, entering the bloodstream immediately, is known as a(n) _____ medication.

7. The generic name of a medication is also known as the _____ name.

8. The strength of a medication is also known as the _____ of that medication.

9. Medication injected into the subcutaneous layer, or fatty tissue, of the skin is known as a(n) _____ injection.

10. A drug has a widespread influence on the body because it is absorbed into the bloodstream; this generalized response to a drug by the body is known as a(n) _____ effect.

11. A rapid heartbeat, over 100 beats per minute, is known as

    a. bradycardia
    b. tachycardia
    c. endocardia
    d. telecardia

12. The dose of a medication that achieves the desired effect is the

    a. therapeutic dose
    b. topical dose
    c. adverse dose
    d. potentiation dose

13. _____ is defined as the body's decreased response to the effect of a drug after repeated dosages.

    a. tolerance
    b. potentiation
    c. potency
    d. side effect

14. Medications available without a prescription are known as

    a. controlled substances
    b. intravenous medications
    c. over-the-counter medications
    d. official drugs

15. An unusual, inappropriate response to a drug or to the usual effective dose of a drug, or a reaction that can be life-threatening, is known as a(n)

    a. desired effect
    b. controlled drug dose
    c. idiosyncrasy
    d. chemotherapy

16. An undesired effect of a medication that occurs within 30 to 90 minutes after administration of the first dose is known as _____ effect. (hint: two words)

17. The effect that occurs when two drugs administered together produce a more powerful response than the sum of their individual effects is known as _____

18. The word element *alges/o* means _____

19. The word element *bi/o* means _____

20. The word element *gloss/o* means _____

G. What Is This?

Read the statements that follow and identify the medication response occurring. Write the most appropriate answer in the space provided.

1. Susan Knight has had a headache for three days, and the medication she has been taking has not relieved the headache. Today she saw her family physician, and he prescribed a medication to relieve her headaches. He indicated that Susan should take two of these pills every four hours as needed for pain. The first dose of this medication was very effective with Susan and achieved the desired effect. She no longer has a headache. The amount of medication that produced this desired effect is known as what dose?

   _____

2. Mr. Jones suffers from kidney disease. He has been taking a medication recently that does not appear to be working properly in his body, and he is feeling worse instead of better. His doctor has run some tests and has determined that the drug is not being completely excreted from the body before another dose is given, so the drug is starting to accumulate in the body tissues, causing the undesired effects. What type of effect of the medication is Mr. Jones experiencing?

   _____

3. Mrs. Smith just received an intramuscular injection of penicillin in the office (she has never had an injection of penicillin before). Within minutes of receiving the injection, Mrs. Smith begins to experience acute respiratory distress, hypotension, edema, tachycardia, cool pale skin, and cyanosis. What type of reaction to the medication is Mrs. Smith experiencing? (hint: two words)

   _____

4. Mr. Brown keeps returning to the doctor, stating that the pain medication he is receiving is not relieving his back pain. He feels that he needs a stronger medication. The doctor has noticed that Mr. Brown has developed a decreased sensitivity to subsequent doses of this pain medication and requires increasingly larger doses to get the full effect of the drug. He plans to try Mr. Brown on a new medication that may be effective. What is the name of Mr. Brown's response to the medication he is currently taking?

   _____

5. Mrs. Monroe has recently begun taking Coumadin, a blood thinner. Today she returned to the doctor for routine testing to make sure the medication is working. The test results revealed that her blood is much thinner than it should be. When questioning Mrs. Monroe, it was discovered that she has also been taking aspirin on a regular basis for general discomfort. The doctor informed Mrs. Monroe that she should not take aspirin while taking Coumadin, because taking these two drugs together will cause a more powerful response in the body than when taking the Coumadin alone. What is the name of Mrs. Monroe's reaction to the two medications taken together?

   _____

H. Spelling

Identify the correct spelling of each medical term. Write the correct spelling in the space provided.

1. antiarrithmic   antiarrhythmic   _____

2. contraindication   contraindiction   _____

3. interavenus   intravenous   _____

4. parential   parenteral   _____

5. sublinugual   sublingual   _____

I. Pronunciation to Spelling

Using the phonetic pronunciations that follow, spell the word correctly. Write your response in the space provided.

1. (**KYOO**-mew-**lay**-shun) _____

2. (jeh-**NAIR**-ik) _____

3. (**id**-ee-oh-**SIN**-krah-see) _____

4. (**in**-trah-**MUSS**-kyoo-lar) _____

5. (sub-**LING**-gwal) _____

J. Match Point

Match the following abbreviations to the appropriate definition.

____ 1. FDA   a. *Physician Desk Reference*

____ 2. FDCA   b. kilogram

____ 3. kg   c. Food Drug and Cosmetic Act

____ 4. mg   d. milligram

____ 5. PDR   e. Food and Drug Administration

K. Construct-a-Word

Using the word elements below, construct words that match the meanings below. Be sure to drop the combining vowel when necessary.

trans-	derm/o	-ia
sub-	pharmac/o	-al
tachy-	toxic/o	-ist
cardi/o	-al	lingu/o
-logy		

1. pertaining to across the skin _____

2. one who is licensed to prepare and dispense drugs _____

3. pertaining to under the tongue _____

4. the study of poisons _____

5. rapid heartbeat, over 100 beats per minute (noun form) _____

L. Is It the Same?

Read each question carefully and provide the most appropriate response. Record your response in the space provided.

1. Does *brand name* mean the same as *trade name*?

   _____ Yes   _____ No

   If "No," which word means "the name under which the drug is sold by a specific manufacturer"?

   _____

2. Does *local effect* mean same as *systemic effect*?

   _____ Yes   _____ No

   If "No," which word means "response (to a medication) confined to a specific part of the body"?

   _____

3. Does *official name* mean the same as *generic name*?

   _____ Yes   _____ No

   If "No," which word means "the name established when the drug is first manufactured"?

   _____

4. Does *initial dose* mean the same as *first dose*?

   _____ Yes   _____ No

   If "No," which word means "the first dose of a medication"?

   _____

5. Does *sublingual medication* mean the same as *buccal medication*?

   _____ Yes   _____ No

   If "No," which word means "a medication that is placed in the mouth next to the cheek"?

   _____

CHAPTER 23

Mental Health

A. Review Checkpoint: Defense Mechanisms

Completion: Read each statement carefully and write the appropriate answer in the space provided.

1. The defense mechanism _____ is an effort to overcome, or make up for, real or imagined inadequacies, as in making up for a deficiency in physical size by excelling in academics.

2. The defense mechanism _____ is the refusal to admit or acknowledge the reality of something, thus avoiding emotional conflict or anxiety, as in a child refusing to admit that he or she is being abused by a parent.

3. The defense mechanism _____ is the process of transferring a feeling or emotion from the original idea or object to a substitute idea or object, as in an individual is angry at the boss but cannot express that anger; the feelings are transferred by criticizing everyone else.

4. The defense mechanism _____ is attempting to make excuses or invent logical reasons to justify unacceptable feelings or behaviors, as in a student making excuses that he or she failed a test because the questions were too confusing.

5. The defense mechanism _____ is a response to stress in which the individual reverts to an earlier level of development and the comfort measures associated with that level of functioning, as in a child may revert to an earlier stage of development, such as bed-wetting, when confronted with a stress in his or her life (such as a new baby in the family).

B. Review Checkpoint: Vocabulary

Build-a-Word: Test your word building skills. Using the clues below, build the appropriate medical terms.

1. Build a word that means "lack of or loss of appetite, resulting in the inability to eat."

   _____ + _____ = _____
     prefix   suffix   word

2. Build a word that means "a sense of well-being or elation (good emotional state)."

   _____ + _____ = _____
     prefix   suffix   word

3. Build a word that means "a sexual disorder in which the individual is sexually aroused and engages in sexual activity with children, generally age 13 or younger (attraction to children)."

   _____ + _____ + _____ = _____
    word root   vowel   suffix   word

4. Build a word that means "a physician who specializes in the diagnosis, prevention, and treatment of mental disorders (one who treats the mind)."

   _____ + _____ = _____
    word root   suffix   word

5. Build a word that means "pertaining to the expression of an emotional conflict through physical symptoms (pertaining to the body and the mind)."

	+		+		+		=	
word root		vowel		word root		suffix		word

C. Review Checkpoint: Word Elements

Matching: Match the word elements listed on the left to the appropriate definition on the right.

_____ 1. -iatrist   a. self

_____ 2. -mania   b. abnormal fear

_____ 3. phil/o   c. madness

_____ 4. -phobia   d. one who treats; a physician

_____ 5. aut/o   e. attraction to

D. Review Checkpoint: Mental Disorders

Completion: Read each statement carefully and write the appropriate answer in the space provided.

1. A progressive, organic mental disorder characterized by chronic personality disintegration, confusion, disorientation, stupor, deterioration of intellectual capacity and function, and impairment of control of memory, judgment, and impulses is known as _____.

2. A(n) _____ disorder is a psychological disorder characterized by episodes of mania and depression, alternations between the two, or a mixture of the two moods simultaneously.

3. A(n) _____ disorder is characterized by recurrent panic attacks that come on unexpectedly, followed by at least one month of persistent concern about having another attack.

4. A sleep disorder characterized by a repeated, uncontrollable desire to sleep—often several times a day—is known as _____.

5. _____ is a condition of persistent inattention and hyperactivity, impulsivity, or both. It is a condition that becomes obvious in some children in the preschool and early school years. (hint: four words)

E. Review Checkpoint: Treatments and Therapies

Matching: Match the treatment/therapy on the left to the appropriate definition on the right.

_____ 1. family therapy

_____ 2. hypnosis

_____ 3. play therapy

_____ 4. psychoanalysis

_____ 5. behavior therapy

a. a form of psychotherapy that analyzes the individual's unconscious thought, using free association, questioning, probing, and analyzing

b. a form of psychotherapy in which a child plays in a protected and structured environment with games and toys provided by a therapist, who observes the behavior, effect, and conversation of the child to gain insights into thoughts, feelings, and fantasies

c. a passive, trancelike state of existence that resembles normal sleep during which perception and memory are altered, resulting in increased responsiveness to suggestion

   d. a form of psychotherapy that seeks to modify observable, maladjusted patterns of behavior, substituting new responses to given stimuli

   e. a form of psychotherapy that focuses the treatment on the process between family members that supports and sustains symptoms

F. Review Checkpoint: Common Abbreviations

Completion: Read the abbreviations below and write the meaning in the space provided.

1. ADD _____

2. MA _____

3. IQ _____

4. TAT _____

5. MMPI _____

G. Review Checkpoint: Putting It All Together

The following questions offer a review of the material studied in the chapter on mental health. Read each question carefully and select or write the most appropriate answer.

1. The voluntary blocking of unpleasant feelings and experiences from one's mind is known as

  a. suppression
  b. regression
  c. sublimation
  d. repression

2. The absence or suppression of observable emotions, feelings, concerns, or passions is known as

  a. delirium
  b. mania
  c. apathy
  d. effect

3. An uncontrolled craving for food, often resulting in eating binges, followed by vomiting to eliminate the food from the stomach; also characterized by the individual feeling depressed, going through a period of self-deprivation, followed by another eating binge, and the cycle continuing, is known as

  a. cataplexy
  b. bulimia nervosa
  c. anxiety disorder
  d. anorexia nervosa

4. An acute and sometimes fatal psychotic reaction caused by cessation of excessive intake of alcoholic beverages over a long period of time is known as

  a. cyclothymic disorder
  b. cataplexy
  c. delirium tremens
  d. amnesia

5. A disorder (seen primarily in adolescent girls) characterized by an emotional disturbance concerning body image, prolonged refusal to eat followed by extreme weight loss, amenorrhea, and a lingering, abnormal fear of becoming obese, is known as

  a. cataplexy
  b. bulimia nervosa
  c. anxiety disorder
  d. anorexia nervosa

6. A willful and deliberate faking of symptoms of a disease or injury to gain some consciously desired end is known as _____.

7. _____ is the means of ridding the body of what has been consumed; that is, the individual may induce vomiting or use laxatives to rid the body of food that has just been eaten.

8. The fear of high places that results in extreme anxiety is known as _____.

9. A morbid fear of fresh air or drafts is known as _____.

10. _____ is an abnormal fear of being in an open, crowded, or public place (such as a field, congested street, or busy department store) where escape may be difficult.

11. Which of the following terms means "fear of spiders"?

    a. arachnophobia   c. acrophobia
    b. zoophobia   d. agoraphobia

12. The fear of being in, or becoming trapped in enclosed or narrow places (fear of enclosed spaces) is known as

    a. nyctophobia   c. aerophobia
    b. agoraphobia   d. claustrophobia

13. An obsessive, irrational fear of darkness is known as

    a. acrophobia   c. claustrophobia
    b. nyctophobia   d. zoophobia

14. A chronic mood disorder characterized by numerous periods of mood swings from depression to happiness with the period of mood disturbance being at least two years in duration is known as

    a. paranoid schizophrenia   c. phobic disorder
    b. panic disorder   d. cyclothymic disorder

15. A(n) _____ disorder is one in which the individual represses anxiety experienced by emotional conflicts by converting the anxious feelings into physical symptoms that have no organic basis but are perceived to be real by the individual.

    a. conversion   c. major depressive
    b. anxiety   d. phobic

16. A somewhat rare form of child abuse in which a parent of a child falsifies an illness in a child by fabricating or creating the symptoms and then seeks frequent medical attention for the child is known as

    a. hypochondriasis   c. Munchausen syndrome (by proxy)
    b. narcolepsy   d. pedophilia

17. _____ is the sexual disorder involving the exposure of one's genitals to a stranger.

18. _____ personality disorder is characterized by a generalized distrust and suspiciousness of others so much so that the individual blames them for his or her own mistakes and feelings.

19. _____ is the term used for education offered to individuals who live with a psychological disturbance.

20. The _____ is determined by dividing the mental age (MA) by the chronological age (CA) and multiplying the result by 100.

H. What Is This?

Read the statements that follow and identify the behavior therapy described. Write the appropriate answer in the space provided.

1. The therapist is treating Ms. Quan for panic disorder. She is using a form of psychotherapy that seeks to modify observable, maladjusted patterns of behavior by substituting new responses to given stimuli. The therapist is striving to change Ms. Quan's feelings of fear and panic to a belief that she is able to master the situation. What is the name of this therapy?

   _____

2. The therapist has been working with Mr. Rockford to overcome his dependence on alcohol. As part of his treatment, the therapist plans to use a form of psychotherapy that focuses the treatment on the process between family members that supports and sustains symptoms. He will focus on validating the importance of each member in the family, concentrating on the fact that the problem is a "family" problem—not just an individual's problem. Hopefully, his therapy will lead the family members toward focusing on ways to solve the central conflict within the family. What is the name of this therapy?

   _____

3. Ms. Woodbury was a recent victim of a crime and cannot remember the details. The police need more details that will assist them in their search for the criminal. Her therapist feels he can help her remember by using a form of psychotherapy that involves placing Ms. Woodbury in a passive, trancelike state of existence that resembles normal sleep during which perception and memory are altered, resulting in increased responsiveness to suggestion. While Ms. Woodbury is in this trancelike state of existence, the therapist may direct her to remember some of the forgotten events of the crime. What is the name of this form of therapy?

   _____

4. Ms. White has been having behavior problems with her four-year-old daughter. Her daughter has been in a new day care center for the last six months, as Ms. White has recently returned to work full time. She has tried numerous things to improve the inappropriate behaviors she is observing in her daughter. After many attempts and no real success, Ms. White has taken her daughter to a psychotherapist. Today, the therapist is utilizing a form of psychotherapy in which the child will play in a protected and structured environment with games and toys provided by the therapist. During this session, the therapist will observe the behavior, affect, and conversation of the child to gain insight into thoughts, feelings, and fantasies of the child. The therapist will help Ms. White's daughter work through any conflicts discovered during the session. What is the name of this form of therapy?

   _____

5. The therapist is seeing a patient today who is being treated for severe depression that has not responded to drug treatment. The therapist is using a process of passing an electrical current through the brain to create a brief seizure in the brain, much like a spontaneous seizure from some form of epilepsy. After properly preparing the patient, a small electric current lasting no longer than a second passes through two electrodes that have been placed on the individual's head. The current excites the nerve tissue and stimulates a brain seizure that lasts from 60 to 90 seconds. Upon awakening after the procedure, the individual usually has no conscious memory of the treatment. Positive results are usually seen after several treatments, as evidenced by the reduction of depression. What is the name of this form of therapy?

   _____

I. Spelling

Identify the correct spelling of each medical term. Write the correct spelling in the space provided

1. hypnosus   hypnosis   _____

2. malingering   melingering   _____

3. neurosis   nuereosis   _____

4. paranoia   paranoy   _____

5. psychotrophic   psychotropic   _____

J. Pronunciation to Spelling

Using the phonetic pronunciations that follow, spell the word correctly. Write your response in the space provided.

1. (an-oh-**REK**-see-ah) _____

2. (dee-**MEN**-shee-ah) _____

3. (pair-ah-**NOY**-ah) _____

4. (**sigh**-koh-**AN**-ah-list) _____

5. (rih-**PRESH**-un) _____

K. Construct-a-Word

Using the word elements below, construct words that match the meanings below. Be sure to drop the combining vowel when necessary.

an-	ped/o	-orexia
eu-	psych/o	-phoria
narc/o	-philia	-logy
-lepsy		

1. loss of appetite _____

2. a sense of well-being or elation _____

3. a sexual disorder in which the individual is sexually aroused and engages in sexual activity with children (age 13 or younger) _____

4. the study of behavior and the processes of the mind _____

5. a sleep disorder characterized by a repeated, uncontrolled desire to sleep _____

L. Is It the Same?

Read each question carefully and provide the most appropriate response. Record your response in the space provided.

1. Does *repression* mean the same as *suppression*?

   _____ Yes   _____ No

   If "No," which word means "the voluntary blocking of unpleasant feelings and experiences from one's mind"?

   _____

2. Does *dysphoria* mean the same as *euphoria*?

   _____ Yes   _____ No

   If "No," which word means "a sense of well-being or elation"?

   _____

3. Does *marijuana* mean the same as *cannabis*?

   _____ Yes   _____ No

   If "No," which word means "a mind-altering drug derived from the flowering top of hemp plants"?

   _____

4. Does *paraphilia* mean the same as *pedophilia*?

   _____ Yes   _____ No

   If "No," which word means "a sexual disorder in which the individual is sexually aroused and engages in sexual activity with children (age 13 or younger)"?

   _____

5. Does *projection* mean the same as *introjection*?

   _____ Yes   _____ No

   If "No," which word means "the transferring of one's own unacceptable thoughts or feelings to someone else"?

   _____

Gerontology

A. Review Checkpoint: Vocabulary

Build-a-Word: Test your word building skills. Using the clues below, build the appropriate medical terms.

1. Build a word that means "without appetite."

   _____ + _____ = _____
     prefix   suffix   word

2. Build a word that means "the surgical removal of a bunion."

   _____ + _____ = _____
    word root   suffix   word

3. Build a word that means "elevated blood sugar level."

   _____ + _____ + _____ = _____
     prefix   word root   suffix   word

4. Build a word that means "poor vision due to aging."

   _____ + _____ = _____
    word root   suffix   word

5. Build a word that means "pertaining to old age."

   _____ + _____ = _____
    word root   suffix   word

B. Review Checkpoint: Word Elements

Matching: Match the word elements listed on the left to the appropriate definition on the right.

____ 1. glauc/o   a. sugar

____ 2. geront/o   b. retina

____ 3. retin/o   c. stiff

____ 4. ankyl/o   d. gray, silver

____ 5. glyc/o   e. old age

C. Review Checkpoint: Pathological Conditions

Completion: Read each statement carefully and write the appropriate answer in the space provided.

1. An acrochordon (cutaneous papilloma) is a benign growth that hangs from a short stalk, commonly occurring on the neck, eyelids, axilla, or groin of an older person, and is also known as a(n) _____. (hint: two words)

2. This condition literally means "porous bones" (that is, bones that were once strong become fragile due to loss of bone density) and is known as _____.

3. Men between the ages of 40 and 60 are more commonly affected by _____, a metabolic disorder characterized by inflammation of the first metatarsal joint of the great toe.

4. Older adults often experience _____ (although it is not limited to this age group), a condition of the legs involving annoying sensations of uneasiness, tiredness, itching, or tingling of the leg muscles while resting. (hint: three words)

5. _____ frequently affects the older population as a result of aging and results in a "turning in" of the eyelash margins (especially the lower margins), resulting in the sensation similar to that of a foreign body in the eye.

D. Review Checkpoint: Diagnostic Techniques, Treatments, and Procedures

Completion: Read each statement carefully and write the appropriate answer in the space provided.

1. The oral administration of a radiopaque contrast medium, barium sulfate, which flows into the esophagus as the person swallows, is known as a(n) _____. (hint: two words)

2. A(n) _____ is the surgical removal of the anterior segment of the lens capsule and the lens of the eye, allowing for insertion of an intraocular lens implant. (hint: three words)

3. The surgical removal of the prostate gland by making an incision into the abdominal wall, just above the pubis, is known as a(n) _____. (hint: two words)

4. The treatment of choice for a fractured hip is usually surgery. Devices such as screws, pins, wires, and nails may be used to internally maintain the bone alignment while healing takes place. These devices are known as _____ devices. (hint: two words)

5. _____ are devices that amplify sound to provide more precise perception and interpretation of words communicated to the individual with a hearing deficit. (hint: two words)

E. Review Checkpoint: Common Abbreviations

Completion: Read the abbreviations below and write the meaning in the space provided.

1. BPH _____

2. CVD _____

3. ADL _____

4. CHF _____

5. AD _____

F. Review Checkpoint: Putting It All Together

The following questions offer a review of the material studied in the chapter on gerontology. Read each question carefully and select or write the most appropriate answer.

1. Which of the following terms means "partial or complete loss of hair"?

   a. alopecia
   b. ascites
   c. bruit
   d. crepitation

2. Which of the following terms means "cramplike pains in the calves of the legs caused by poor circulation to the muscles of the legs"?

   a. crepitation
   b. claudication
   c. dyskinesia
   d. atrophy

3. Which of the following terms means "clicking or crackling sounds heard upon joint movement"?

   a. crepitation
   b. claudication
   c. dyskinesia
   d. atrophy

4. Which of the following terms means "thickening and hardening of the skin"?

   a. myopia
   b. lichenification
   c. kyphosis
   d. entropion

5. Which of the following terms can be checked by lightly pinching the skin of the forearm between the examiner's thumb and forefinger, indicating a reflection of the skin's elasticity?

   a. turgor
   b. lichenification
   c. acrochordon
   d. senile lentigines

6. The word element *arthr/o* means _____.

7. The word element *geront/o* means _____.

8. The word element *-opia* means _____.

9. The word element *spondyl/o* means _____.

10. The word element *-uria* means _____.

11. Which of the following terms refers to the process of growing old?

    a. lichenification
    b. crepitation
    c. senescence
    d. dyskinesia

12. Which of the following terms means "loss of hearing due to the natural aging process"?

    a. presbycusis
    b. presbyopia
    c. Presbyterian
    d. microtia

13. Which of the following terms means "loss of accommodation for near vision—poor vision due to the natural aging process"?

    a. presbycusis
    b. presbyopia
    c. Presbyterian
    d. myopia

14. Which of the following terms is used to describe an individual between the ages of 75 and 84 years?

    a. old-old
    b. young-old
    c. middle-old
    d. senescence

15. Which of the following terms is used to describe an individual between the ages of 65 and 74?

    a. old-old
    b. young-old
    c. middle-old
    d. senescence

16. A fracture of the hip is a break in the continuity of the bone involving the upper third of the _____.

17. The condition that occurs most frequently in postmenopausal women, in which bones that were once strong become fragile due to loss of bone density, is known as _____.

18. An abnormal enlargement of the joint at the base of the great toe is known as _____.

19. Degenerative joint disease is also known as _____.

20. _____ disease is a progressive, degenerative disease that affects the cortex of the brain and begins with minor memory loss and progresses to complete loss of mental, emotional, and physical functioning.

G. What Is This?

Read the statements that follow and identify the diagnostic technique, treatment, or procedure described. Write the appropriate answer in the space provided.

1. Mr. Gilmore recently had a test that revealed some blockages in his coronary arteries. He has been admitted to the hospital for a surgical procedure designed to increase the blood flow to the myocardial muscle. Grafts made from veins taken from other parts of the body (usually the saphenous vein from the leg) will be connected to the coronary artery above and below the occlusion. The connection will join the two vessels, restoring the normal flow of oxygenated blood to the myocardium. What is the name of this surgery? (hint: four words)

   _____

2. Mrs. Kirby has type 2 diabetes and has experienced some recent retinal bleeding. Her ophthalmologist has scheduled her for a surgical procedure that uses an argon laser to treat diabetic retinopathy. The argon laser will be used to seal microaneurysms and to reduce the risk of hemorrhage. What is the name of this procedure? (hint: two words)

   _____

3. Mr. McGee suffers from benign prostatic hypertrophy. The condition has not responded to conservative measures. His urologist has scheduled him for the surgical removal of the prostate gland. The physician will be making an incision into Mr. McGee's abdominal wall, just above the pubis. A small incision will then be made into the bladder (which will be distended with fluid) and the prostate gland will be removed through the bladder cavity. What is the name of this surgical procedure? (hint: two words)

   _____

4. Mr. Robinson is suffering from a cataract of the left eye. His ophthalmologist has scheduled him for surgery to remove the anterior segment of the lens capsule and the lens, allowing for the insertion of an intraocular lens implant. What type of cataract extraction is this?

   _____

5. Mrs. Hunt has been complaining of unexplained rectal bleeding. Her physician has scheduled her for a procedure that involves an infusion of a radiopaque contrast medium, barium sulfate, into the rectum, to be held in place in the lower intestinal tract while X-ray films are obtained of the lower GI tract. The physician will be checking for possible abnormal findings such as malignant tumors, colonic fistula, and/or polyps. What is the name of this procedure?

   _____

H. Spelling

Identify the correct spelling of each medical term. Write the correct spelling in the space provided.

1. anorexia   anorexa   _____
2. claudacation   claudication   _____
3. crepidtation   crepitation   _____
4. curretage   curettage   _____
5. turgor   turger   _____

I. Pronunciation to Spelling

Using the phonetic pronunciations that follow, spell the word correctly. Write your response in the space provided.

1. (al-oh-**PEE**-she-ah) _____
2. (ak-roh-**KOR**- don) _____
3. (jer-ee-**AT**-riks) _____
4. (seh-**NESS**-ens) _____
5. (**jer**-on-**TOL**-oh-jee) _____

J. Match Point

Match the following abbreviations to the appropriate definition.

____ 1. CAD   a. gerontological nurse practitioner
____ 2. URI   b. stroke
____ 3. GNP   c. coronary artery disease
____ 4. TIA   d. upper respiratory infection
____ 5. CVA   e. transient ischemic attack

K. Construct-a-Word

Using the word elements that follow, construct words that match the meanings below. Be sure to drop the combining vowel when necessary.

a-	troph/o	-ic
	geront/o	-opia
	noct/o	-phobia
	geront/o	-uria
	presby/o	-ics

1. characterized by a wasting away of tissues _____
2. pertaining to old age _____
3. an abnormal fear of growing old _____
4. urination at night _____
5. poor vision due to the aging process _____

L. Is It the Same?

Read each question carefully and provide the most appropriate response. Record your response in the space provided.

1. Does *osteoarthritis* mean the same as *degenerative joint disease*?

   _____ Yes   _____ No

   If "No," which word means "arthritis that results from wear and tear on the joints, especially weight-bearing joints such as the hips and knees"?

   _____

2. Does *ectropion* mean the same as *entropion*?

   _____ Yes   _____ No

   If "No," which word means "'turning inward' of the eyelash margins (especially the lower margins)"?

   _____

3. Does *cataract* mean the same as *glaucoma*?

   _____ Yes   _____ No

   If "No," which word means "the lens in the eye becomes progressively cloudy, losing its normal transparency"?

   _____

4. Does *gerontophobia* mean the same as *senescence*?

   _____ Yes   _____ No

   If "No," which word means "the process of growing old"?

   _____

5. Does *acrochordon* mean the same as *skin tag*?

   _____ Yes   _____ No

   If "No," which word means "a benign growth that hangs from a short stalk, commonly occurring on the neck, eyelids, axilla, or groin"?

   _____